EAT *Yourself* BEAUTIFUL

TRUE BEAUTY, FROM THE INSIDE OUT

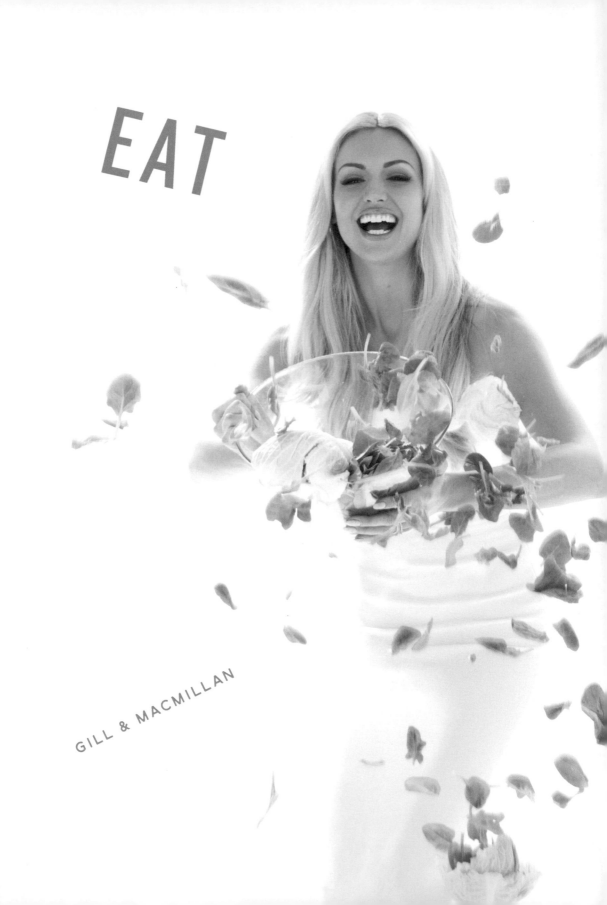

EAT

GILL & MACMILLAN

YOURSELF

BEAUTIFUL

True beauty, from the inside out

ROSANNA DAVISON

GILL & MACMILLAN

Hume Avenue
Park West
Dublin 12
www.gillmacmillanbooks.ie

978 07171 6699 2

Design by www.grahamthew.com
Food photography by Neil Hurley
Photos on pp. ii, vi, 13, 25, 42 and 60 © Barry McCall
Photos on p. 6 courtesy of Rosanna Davison
Food styling by Anne Marie Tobin, assisted by Frances Halpin
Edited by Kristin Jensen
Indexed by Cliff Murphy
Printed by Printer Trento Srl, Italy

This book is typeset in 10.5 on 13pt Neutra Text.

The paper used in this book comes from the wood pulp of managed forests.
For every tree felled, at least one tree is planted, thereby renewing natural
resources.

A CIP catalogue record for this book is available from the British Library.

54321

ACKNOWLEDGEMENTS

I would like to start by thanking Conor, Catherine and all at
Gill & Macmillan for their support and belief in me.

Thank you to my wonderful lecturers at the College of Naturopathic Medicine
for educating me and firing up my passion for nutrition and health.
I'm so thankful for the amazing support from my wonderful family and friends,
and especially my parents, Chris and Diane, for their invaluable
advice and encouragement.

Finally, the most special thanks goes to my husband, Wesley, for his
unwavering patience, support and encouragement throughout the many
hours, days, weeks and months that I worked hard on this book.
I'm incredibly grateful!

Rosanna x

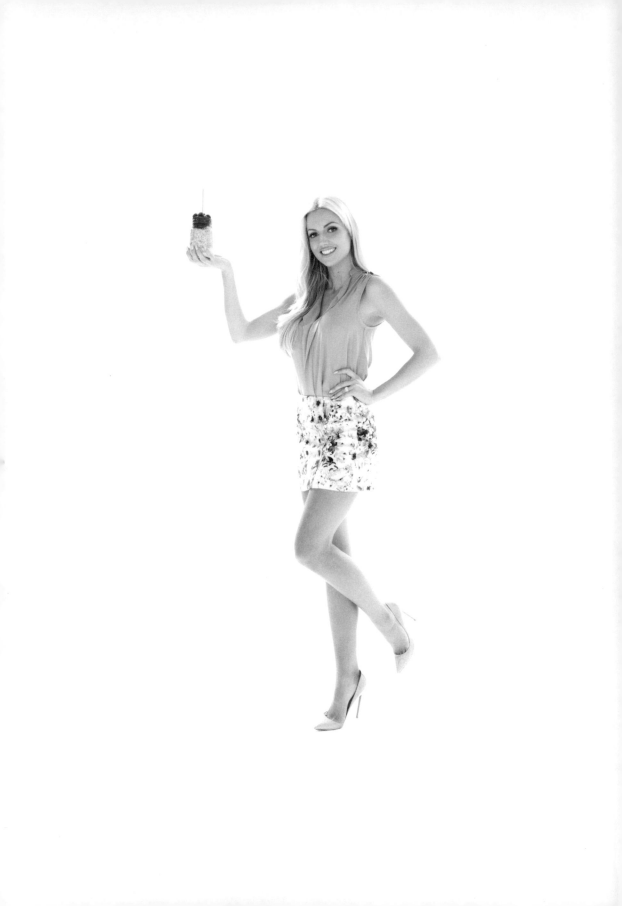

CONTENTS

PREFACE

THE IDEA FOR *EAT YOURSELF BEAUTIFUL* was born from the hundreds of beauty and fitness questions I've been asked over the past 12 years as an international model. My career began when I was crowned Miss World in southern China in 2003 at the age of 19. Being immersed in an industry so obsessed with outward appearance, I fully believed that the various lotions, creams and serums I smeared on my face, hair and body were the key to glowing skin, luscious locks and eternal youth. The many make-up artists, hair stylists and other beauty professionals I worked with would excitedly talk about the outstanding benefits of whatever miracle products were the current cult favourites being touted by the racks of girly mags in every newsagent. So of course I bought into it all and spent a small fortune. I didn't know any better and I believed the hype.

Beauty products do have their place and can make a big difference to our appearance and self-confidence. But much like the drugs of modern medicine, they tend to cover up any issues or symptoms rather than get to the source of the problem. As a teenager and in my early 20s, I spent many nights covering my spots with a blob of Sudocrem without thinking about why I was getting persistent pimples in the first place. It didn't occur to me that an internal imbalance might be causing my breakouts. It was only when I began my training as a nutritional therapist in 2010 that I began to study and really understand the inner workings of the human body, a magnificent creation. It dawned on me that we literally are what we eat. Eating your vegetables to grow up big and strong isn't just a line repeated to us by frustrated parents at the dinner table. It's really true! As our biggest organ, our skin is a true reflection of the internal health of our body, and who doesn't want healthy, glowing, beautiful skin?

I have answered so many questions from all sorts of people about the secrets to good skin, hair, nails, energy and weight loss. They all want to know what products to buy, what foundation is best for a perfect complexion and how to lose weight without feeling hungry. And my answer is simple: your diet is the best beauty secret you possess. You are in control of everything that goes into your body. All you need is a little time and patience to allow your body to heal and reap the numerous benefits of my tried and trusted way of eating, designed to give you the body, skin and hair you have always dreamed of. Best of all, it really isn't complicated.

I understand how intimidating it can be to navigate the seemingly endless world of nutrition brands, superfoods, supplement powders, vitamin pills, high-protein diets, low-carb diets, fat and weight loss, so I have explained it all for you in this book. Whether you eat meat or just plants, are watching the pennies or are happy to spend, my advice suits every taste, budget and lifestyle. This isn't about restriction. I don't count calories or ever go hungry, and I don't expect you to either. My food and health philosophy is all about eating high-quality, nutrient-dense foods that nourish your body and help to regulate your appetite, weight, hormones and cravings naturally. You will be feeling fully satisfied and bursting with health, vitality and boundless energy.

I hope you enjoy reading this book as much as I have enjoyed writing it. It's a true work of love and the result of many years spent on a food and health journey. I've made my fair share of mistakes and have asked more questions than I've answered at times, but it has been absolutely worth it. I am delighted to share this journey with you as you bring out your most beautiful self.

In beautiful health,

Rosanna x

INTRODUCTION: MY STORY

'THE FOOD YOU EAT CAN BE EITHER THE
SAFEST AND MOST POWERFUL FORM OF
MEDICINE OR THE SLOWEST FORM OF
POISON.' *Ann Wigmore*

AS A LITTLE GIRL, my family called me 'the cream monster'. I was utterly in love with the taste and texture of whipped cream and ate it on everything from my grand-mother's homemade treacle tarts and apple pies to bowls of crackling Rice Krispies and even with a side of gravy, mash and peas! At least I was an active child and my mum made sure we ate a healthy diet most of the time, with plenty of home-grown fruit and vegetables. At that age, I naturally had no idea of the impact of nutrition on the human body.

For most people, food serves two purposes: it should taste good and it should fill you up, providing energy. Big multinational food and drink corporations have made billions selling us taste and energy. Indeed, food *should* tick those boxes. Food that doesn't taste good won't exactly fly off the shelves. But the most important purpose of food is nourishment. The trillions of cells in our bodies all rely on certain nutrients to be delivered to them every single day via our bloodstream to help keep us alive. You literally are what you eat.

I clearly remember the first time I made the connection between what was on my plate and what my body was made from, and it was drawn from my lifelong love of animals.

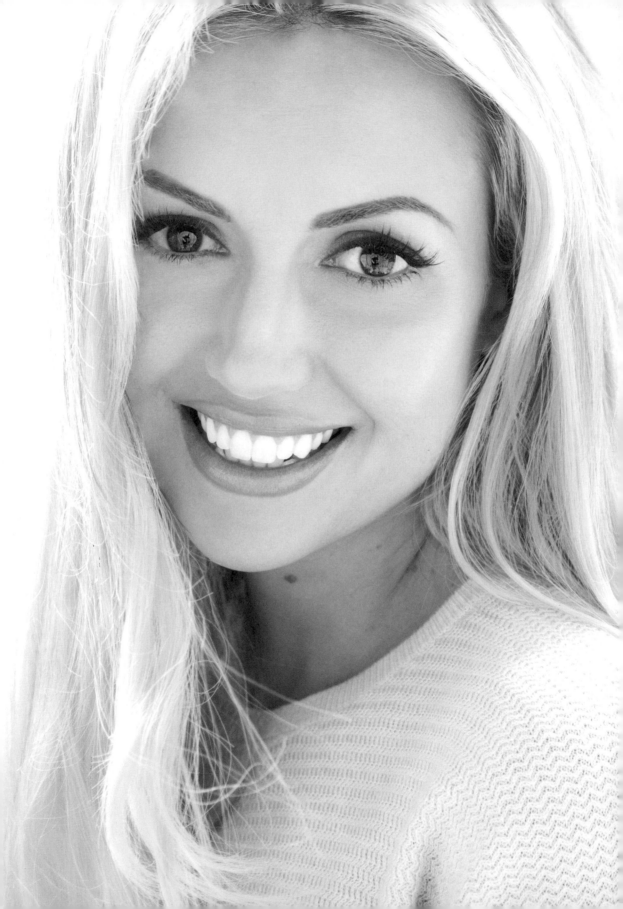

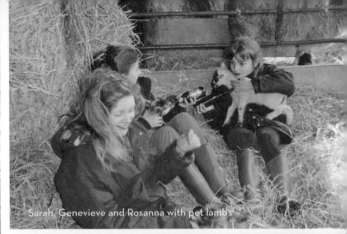
Sarah, Genevieve and Rosanna with pet lambs

Rosanna and dog Milly

Rosanna with granny Maeve Davison,
brothers Hubie and Michael and dog
Milly in 1995

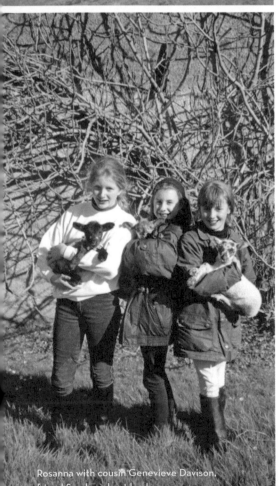
Rosanna with cousin Genevieve Davison,
friend Sarah and pet lambs

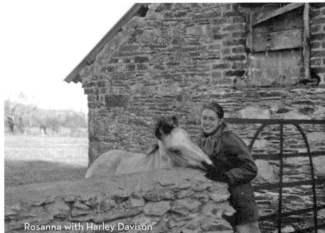
Rosanna with Harley Davison

My wonderful grandmother Maeve Davison, a former spy in the Cold War (yes, really!) and now a retired farmer, used to own a large flock of sheep. Each Easter, my parents brought me and my two younger brothers to her Wexford farm for a week or two, where we would help out with lambing season. All the heavily pregnant ewes were housed in a large barn, each in a spacious pen with a cosy straw bed, which we dubbed The Shepherd's Hotel. With the help of the farmhand, I used to get stuck in with the lambing, rolling up my sleeves and pulling out a tiny squealing newborn. Bringing a new life into the world was a magical feeling. Some lambs were either rejected by their mothers or were orphaned if their mum died during the birth, so I was always given a number of lambs to care for in the first few weeks of their lives. A few times a day, I would prepare bottles of warm milk to hand-feed to the newborns.

One Sunday, I was called in for lunch with the family. Sitting down at the big country kitchen table, I was handed a large plate of roast lamb. I remember staring at the plate and then looking down at my own body, thinking that I'd just spent a couple of hours hand-feeding this tiny creature, and then I was expected to eat one, which would then become part of my own body. For an 11-year-old girl, it was a big moment of realisation. I pushed the plate away and haven't eaten red meat since.

It was an ethical decision, but it ignited my interest in the huge effect that food has on how you look and feel. While I always ate the vegetarian option at school, I did eat chicken at home from time to time. But it just never felt right and I became completely vegetarian at the age of 19. Going vegetarian meant that I had to find more creative ways to eat in a family of meat-eaters, so I started cooking for myself and experimenting in the kitchen. I began eating a lot more raw and steamed salads and vegetables, legumes, nuts and seeds and goat's cheese. I read all about what nutrients vegetarians need and even swapped my cow's milk for calcium-fortified plant milk.

I noticed a big improvement in my immune system first. I used to suffer from regular colds, sore throats and sniffles, but these started becoming more and more rare. Next, I found that my body became leaner and stronger. I did a lot of Pilates at that stage, but abs started popping up where they hadn't been before. My pesky teenage spots also cleared up and my hair grew longer, thicker and shinier. I felt great! But I still knew little about the process of change and healing that my body was going through.

Worried about my iron and calcium intake, my mum sent me to a Dublin dietician, who insisted that I must drink three servings of milk a day to ensure I was getting enough calcium. For the next week I did as I was told, pouring milk on my cereal in the morning, drinking cappuccinos and glasses of milk and eating pots of plain yoghurt. By the end of the week, I had a blocked nose, a big bloated stomach and I had broken out in little white pimples all over my face. The effect it had on me came as quite a surprise. Wasn't milk supposed to do a body good? So once again I reverted to plant milk and for the next few years I really enjoyed the increased energy, vitality and improved immunity as a vegetarian.

In my mid-twenties, I discovered the benefits of weight training and put myself on a high-protein, low-carb diet, convinced that it was the best eating plan for my new exercise regime. I ate this way for about six months but felt increasingly lethargic. I used to rely on black coffee, drink whey protein shakes and eat protein bars and egg whites, thinking that I would become lean and toned. But I actually started to look bloated and began to feel extremely worn out.

By this stage, I had started the first year of my three-year nutrition course. I began to learn about human biochemistry and the effects that foods have on our body at a cellular and hormonal level. I was shocked at what I was learning about the effects of dairy and excess animal protein on our health. As part of a college project, we each had to choose a diet to try for a week in order to be able to explain various popular eating plans to future clients. Some of my classmates chose Atkins, the Zone Diet or paleo, but I picked a raw vegan diet. I was apprehensive and expected to feel hungry and miserable all week, but I ate raw fruit and vegetables, nuts and seeds, coconut flesh and nut butters quite liberally for the week and began to feel really good. By the end of the week, my energy levels had improved, I was sleeping better, my eyes and skin looked brighter and I was starting to look leaner too. Initially all of the extra fibre had been a challenge for my digestive system, but it soon adapted. I felt so good, in fact, that I decided to continue for another week. I began to add in some cooked foods like steamed and roasted veggies and quinoa, but I stuck to the whole foods, plant-based lifestyle, high in raw foods and fibre-rich carbohydrates and with moderate levels of plant protein and heart-healthy fats.

The effect that this had on my health, well-being and appearance was profound. Within two weeks, my energy levels were soaring. I no longer felt tired and reliant on caffeine. Despite the fact that I was eating more food than I ever had before and not counting a single calorie, my body began shrinking fast and within three weeks I had gone down an entire dress size without even trying. My eyes began to sparkle and my skin looked smoother and fresher than ever before. Fine lines even began to disappear. My body was relishing the huge array of nutrients I had started to feed it. I finally felt that I had found the right type of long-term eating plan for me, one that never left me feeling deprived or hungry.

One of the most incredible benefits of eating a plant-based diet came after about six months, when I noticed a huge sense of calm and mental clarity. I used to be a big worrier as a child and suffered severe stress around exam times. Like a storm cloud clearing, I felt calmer than ever before and it seemed that nothing could rile me. My family noticed the change too. It also improved my athletic performance and recovery time, which greatly helped my training for the 2012 Ironman 70.3 half marathon along Galway Bay, which I ran in well under two hours.

Of course, these are all my own anecdotes and experiences. You will inevitably go through your own series of individual changes when you begin to work towards a way of eating to support your detoxification system and build a stronger, more beautiful body. After all, cosmetics and beauty treatments can only do so much. If you want glowing skin, glossy hair, stronger nails, increased energy, better sleep and to achieve the ideal weight for your body, then the changes must begin from within. What you put into your mouth every single day has the ability to change you and your life profoundly.

I have given you a little insight into my own journey of health, which is now both a deeply ingrained way of life and an ongoing adventure. If you are ready to begin your journey, I am honoured to be your guide.

Are you ready to eat yourself beautiful?

BEAUTY BEGINS FROM WITHIN

'THE CURE OF MANY DISEASES IS UNKNOWN TO PHYSICIANS BECAUSE THEY ARE IGNORANT OF THE WHOLE. FOR THE PART CAN NEVER BE WELL UNLESS THE WHOLE IS WELL.' *Plato*

THE GROWTH OF NATURAL MEDICINE

The field of natural medicine has enjoyed a huge surge in popularity in recent years, making it an extremely exciting area to be a part of. When I began studying nutritional biochemistry, I noticed the lack of understanding amongst my friends and family of the role that food has in making us look, feel and function better. Fast forward almost half a decade and so many more people are paying attention to the type and quality of food that they're eating. Enormous bodies of scientific research now show us that the power to live your whole life free from modern lifestyle diseases such as cancer, heart disease and diabetes starts on your plate.

Functional medicine is about treating illness with natural therapies while focusing on promoting health and well-being. It looks at diet, lifestyle and prevention rather than cure. It sees the patient as a whole rather than as a series of organs and autonomous systems. It also treats the mind and body as connected rather than separate entities and gives the patient the ability to make their own healthcare choices.

The most powerful healing force in the universe is nature itself in its ability to restore and overcome disease. In 1995, Dr Caldwell Esselstyn published his benchmark long-term nutrition study that showed that heart disease in severely ill patients could be halted and reversed by putting them on a low-fat, whole foods, plant-based diet. It demonstrated the self-healing power of the human body under ideal conditions. Since natural medicine is so effective at preventing disease rather than just suppressing symptoms, as modern medicine tends to do, I firmly believe that there is a great need for natural medicine to become more widespread than conventional medicine. There are more natural therapies gaining respect in mainstream medicine now than ever before, as it is clear that scientific evidence of the efficiency of natural medicine is solid.

I will be approaching the body and your health in a holistic way in this book, which may be a little different to the mainstream perspective that you're used to. I will also talk about beauty and health either together or separately, but one is not possible without the other. True beauty from the inside out comes from a healthy and optimally functioning body. Glowing skin, glossy hair and a lean, strong body for life will not be achieved without being in the best health possible.

PLANT-BASED NUTRITION

I write a lot in this book about whole foods, plant-based nutrition and eating, rather than a vegetarian or vegan diet. The word *vegan* in particular can be a loaded word with all sorts of associations and connotations. Vegans have often been targeted in the media and popular culture for being particularly outspoken and proactive about their beliefs. I try not to be like that and tend to only answer a question on nutrition when asked rather than questioning what's on other people's plates. I feel that leading by positive example is the best way to help people to change to a healthier lifestyle. I have successfully encouraged family, friends and clients to consider alternative options for commonly problematic foods like wheat and sugar, as I could see that they were harming their health.

There is so much scientific evidence to support a whole foods, plant-based diet that it could easily fill three books. I will mention the results of some of the most significant studies, which must be the gold standard double-blind and peer-reviewed to be considered of real significance to the world

of nutrition and health research. Large food corporations can and have funded studies that are designed to favour their desired outcome, so it's important to make sure that sources of information are genuinely honest and do not have an ulterior motive.

LOOKING TO EVOLUTION FOR ANSWERS

All animals are categorised as herbivore, omnivore or carnivore based on what they *need* to eat by their very make-up, rather than what they *can* eat in their part of the world. Humans are categorised as omnivores and are known to have evolved as hunter-gatherers. This knowledge is based on the evidence we have, both anatomical and historical. Indeed, our digestive systems are able to cope with meat, but evidence shows that plant foods are far more digestible than animal protein. Rather than looking at the foods we all like to eat in the modern world, it's better to look to the animal kingdom and our evolution for answers. Our closest relative genetically is the primate, which eats primarily fruit, blossoms and leafy greens and a much smaller amount of bark, seeds and insects. We share approximately 99.4% of our DNA sequence with the chimpanzee, more than any other animal in the world.

OUR PHYSICAL MAKE-UP

Human saliva contains the enzyme amylase, which begins the chemical process of breaking down carbohydrates from starch to sugars. As animal protein foods are almost devoid of carbs, this enzyme is designed for digesting plant foods. Moving down the body, our long digestive tract further favours plants. Our stomachs are created by nature to best digest plant foods, as they have a far lower concentration of stomach acid than that of a carnivore. Lions, tigers and other meat-eaters have at least 10 times the level of stomach acid that we do, enabling them to easily digest the high amount of tough meat fibres that comprise their diet. Our liver, an extremely important organ for detoxing our blood, processing the food we eat and synthesising vitamins, is not well able to tolerate uric acid. Uric acid is produced when animal protein is digested and is one of the reasons why animal protein foods are said to be acid-forming when we talk about the acid–alkaline balance for optimal health.

Carnivores' livers, on the other hand, contain urate oxidase, an enzyme needed for the breakdown of uric acid. The carnivorous liver is 15 times more able than a human's liver to break down the uric acid produced from protein metabolism.

Our intestines are about 12 times as long as our trunk. Since plant foods move through our gut much more quickly than meat due to their high fibre content, we need plenty of area for absorbing all of those beneficial vitamins and minerals for our health and beauty. The gorilla, also a natural plant-eater, has a similarly long intestine. In contrast, carnivorous animals have a much shorter intestine. It's only about three times the length of their body so that the meat they eat can speedily move through their system, avoiding toxic build-up and poisons. Just imagine the heat in our intestines and what must happen to the meat a human eats as it slowly moves through that long digestive tract. It begins to putrefy and rot, allowing harmful toxins and acidic by-products to leak into the bloodstream. Nature cleverly designed the gut of lions and tigers to avoid such problems.

Vitamin C helps to build up our immune system, preventing colds and flu. That's just one of the many essential jobs of the vitamin that we all associate with oranges, strawberries and kiwis. Humans must eat enough vitamin C daily for good health. As it's a water-soluble vitamin, it isn't stored in the liver or tissues. While humans must eat plenty of plants daily for their vitamin C, carnivores are designed to make all the vitamin C they need daily in their own bodies.

THE IDEAL HUMAN DIET

Leading nutrition expert and author Dr T. Colin Campbell, who has decades of scientific research behind him, summarised the ideal diet for humans: eat whole, plant-based foods that are as natural as they can possibly be, to include a wide range of vegetables, fruits, beans and legumes, raw nuts and seeds and whole grains. Your body will do the work for you once you're feeding it the most nourishing foods, and the more plant foods you eat, the greater nutritional punch they will pack. There are absolutely no nutrients found in animal products that are not found in abundance in plant foods.

You don't have to become a full vegetarian to enjoy the many benefits of plant-based foods for your beauty, energy, weight management and general health. Your reasons for including meat, poultry and eggs in your diet may be for the taste, convenience, traditional or family reasons. My role is simply to explain why we're designed by nature to favour a diet high in whole plant foods, beginning with our digestive system.

A HEALTHY DIGESTIVE SYSTEM

'Digestion is one of the most delicately balanced of all human and perhaps angelic functions.' MFK Fisher

The phrase 'beauty begins from within' may be mentioned a lot in popular culture, but it couldn't be a more truthful statement when it comes to building the most beautiful you. Achieving clear and glowing skin, strong nails, glossy hair, bundles of energy and your ideal body weight are all deeply dependent

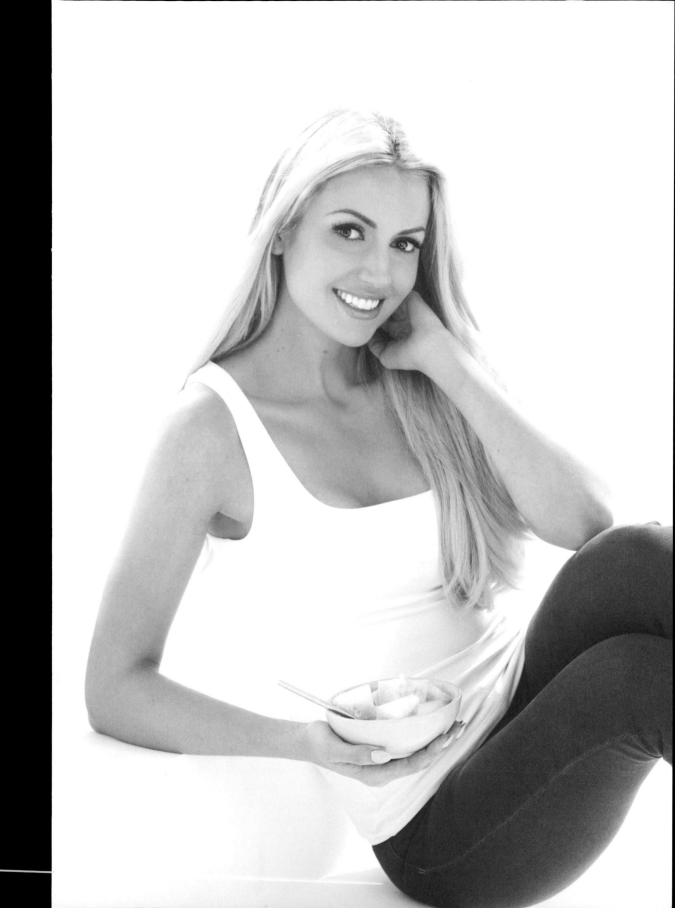

on the health of your digestive system. Your intestines form a barrier between the outside world and your blood, cells, tissues, systems, brain and bones. Your entire body is dependent on the nutrients absorbed through the walls of your gut. To gain the best nutritional benefits from the food you eat, it's essential that it's properly digested, absorbed and eliminated. You could eat the best-quality food in the world, but if you're not absorbing it properly, much of it will be wasted.

You're not what you eat – you're what you absorb! The nutrients from your food must reach every cell in your body to build healthy new cells. The primary job of the gastrointestinal system is to break down and absorb nutrients from food. This process is efficient in humans, as our gut is lined with millions of tiny villi and microvilli contained in circular folds, which are responsible for absorbing the nutrients we eat and enabling absorption by the bloodstream.

Food stays in the stomach from about 45 minutes to four hours, depending on the type of food it is. Fruit takes the least time to digest, while fats and heavy proteins take much longer. No absorption happens in the stomach, apart from simple sugars, alcohol and drugs. That's why booze hits your system so quickly after drinking it and why certain people develop 'beer bellies'.

DIGESTIVE ENERGY

Most of the energy produced in your body each day goes into breaking down your meals and snacks so that you can absorb their nutrients and make more energy for tomorrow's activities. Have you ever felt suddenly woozy and tired after a large, heavy meal, so much so that you needed a short nap? Christmas dinner is notorious for it! Digestion is what can cause your body to age faster and your beauty to diminish, but if treated properly, it can also help you to reach your

highest state of beauty and health for life. The *Eat Yourself Beautiful* plan is designed to maximise your digestive ability, but also to minimise the amount of energy that is used to digest your food so that your energy is *free* to be used in healing your body and regenerating your cells.

The cells in your body are literally made from the food you eat, and how well you absorb your food and the efficiency with which you digest it makes a big difference to the speed at which you will age. Your facial cells, for example, are completely renewed about every month and a half to two months. Most of the cells in your body are totally regenerated within the space of a year. Some cells, such as bones, can take a lot longer to renew themselves, but every seven years we are completely new people, from the top of our heads to the tips of our toes. That's pretty extraordinary! Luckily for us, it also means that if we have had less than ideal health habits in our lives, we can still reverse much of the damage done and heal our body. Years of unhealthy food choices, environmental pollutants, chemicals and preservatives and other toxins gradually build up over time and contribute to the ageing process. Unfortunately, time simply passing also makes a difference to the speed our bodies work at and the ease with which we can maintain weight. As children and teenagers, and even into our twenties, it seems that we can eat what we please and never have to worry. But as time moves on, toxicity and waste can build up in our bodies, making it increasingly difficult to manage our weight, metabolism and energy levels.

Excess weight, puffiness around your eyes, spots, dry skin and hair, brittle nails, poor sleep, low energy and even wrinkles and fine lines can all be rectified when you move towards a more nourishing and healing way of eating and living. There are no magic fixes for optimal health, and perfection is not what should be strived for *all* the time. You need to live a little too! But moving consistently in the right direction is what will make the biggest difference to how you look and feel. It's a lot more cost effective to eat well now than to spend a fortune on treatments, supplements and even doctor appointments in the future.

THE ALKALINE– ACID BALANCE

Following the principles of alkaline eating and maintaining a favourable balance in your cells, tissues and organs is an important aspect of good nutrition and avoiding early ageing, weight gain and disease. Acidity and alkalinity are measured according to the pH scale, which ranges from 0 to 14. With a pH of 7.0, water is neutral. The human body prefers a slightly alkaline pH of between 7.35 and 7.45. All of the food that you eat, when digested, leaves either an acidic or an alkaline residue in your bloodstream, depending on the type of minerals it contains.

It can be hard to know which foods are acidic and which are alkaline because their taste doesn't give much away about what they'll leave in your body once metabolised. Acidic-tasting lemons and limes actually become alkalising once they are broken down in your body. A glass of cow's milk will show up as having an alkaline pH if tested, but when it is digested in your body it leaves a high acidic residue. In fact, all animal products, including dairy, meat, eggs, poultry and fish, leave an acidic residue in your blood. That's just another of the many health risks of popular high-protein diets like Atkins and the Zone Diet.

Using the *Eat Yourself Beautiful* recipes, your body will naturally become flooded with a huge amount of alkaline minerals to cleanse your blood and tissues. But nobody can be perfect all the time, and occasional treats are part of what makes healthy eating more enjoyable. If you do end up eating a large amount of very acidic foods, such as dairy, meat or refined sugar, then your body will be faced with a race against time to maintain its favoured alkaline blood pH before it drops too low. It must prioritise dealing with the sudden rise in blood acidity, which can cause alkaline minerals like calcium to be leached from your skeleton to act as a buffer and return your blood pH back to its preferred alkalinity. Other alkaline minerals, like potassium and magnesium, that help to keep you healthy and beautiful can also be lost or reduced. It's okay to eat some acidic foods, as it can be difficult to always maintain the balance, but your health will flourish and your detoxification system will work best under alkaline conditions.

HEALTHY BONES NEED EXERCISE

Fruit and veggies help to sweep toxic material from your intestines, build clean, nutrient-rich blood and healthy skin, nails and hair. But what actually matters even more for bone health is exercise. Some of us are crazy about all things fitness, while others may have successfully dodged PE throughout school and have no intention of breaking into a sweat these days. But I promise you that one of the single best things you can do for your bones and your overall health and beauty is to move your body. A huge number of studies have clearly shown that physical fitness is a primary determinant of bone density. Just doing one hour of exercise three times a week prevents bone loss and can even increase bone mass in women post-menopause.

Walking, which is simple and free, is one of the very best types of exercise for maintaining healthy bone mass. Others include tennis, dancing, weight lifting and aerobics. I personally love Pilates, weight training and cardiovascular exercise like running and cycling for staying healthy and in shape. The news for those who don't love to exercise is pretty grim, however. A sedentary lifestyle has been shown to result in a significant negative calcium balance through urinary and faecal calcium loss.

RAW FOODS ARE BEAUTY FOODS

When I first changed my entire approach to food and began eating a whole foods, plant-based diet, I included a lot of raw foods. These were mainly veggies, nuts, seeds, coconut, sprouted lentils and beans, and loads of leafy greens. It took some creativity and a different mindset at first, but now I naturally lean towards raw foods most of the time because I find that they really boost my energy, are easier to digest than cooked foods and I never get that heavy, full feeling after eating. I rarely eat a fully cooked meal without a green salad or some chopped raw veggies first.

Raw foods are best for weight loss, as most are low in calories, fat and sodium and high in water and fibre to keep you feeling full. Aiming to make up to 80% of your diet full of these foods will bring about the very best health and beauty results.

The best type of raw foods you can eat are those grown organically, and the ripest fruit and vegetables contain the most vitamins and enzymes. Frozen raw fruit and vegetables are the next best option if fresh are unavailable, and many of the enzymes and nutrients remain intact if they're frozen soon after they're picked.

SPROUTED FOODS

I'm a big fan of sprouting seeds, beans, legumes and grains in a sprouting jar on my kitchen windowsill. They're teeming with enzymes, essential vitamins, minerals and all the nutrients needed for a plant to grow, which is why they're so beneficial to us. Sprouts are also extremely alkaline, fibre rich and full of chlorophyll for healthy, oxygenated blood. I love to eat a big handful of them in a raw wrap for lunch or mix them into salads. Some people have trouble digesting beans, but raw sprouted beans are much easier to digest due to their living enzyme content.

LIVING ENZYMES

Many nutrition and natural medicine experts recommend including as many raw foods in your diet as possible because the living enzymes naturally present in raw food actually lend themselves to the digestive process in your body. Raw nuts, for instance, contain enzymes that help them to be digested in your body, but in roasted nuts, those enzymes become denatured and then die. Eating raw foods means that your system doesn't have to provide all of the enzymes needed for digestion itself. This is great news for building your health and beauty. Energy is freed up to work on other areas of your body, like repairing damaged skin cells.

The foods I recommend in the *Eat Yourself Beautiful* plan are full of the minerals needed in almost all of your body's biochemical processes. Enzymes are important because they act as the stimulant for hundreds of different reactions in your body, such as the creation of collagen to keep skin firm, plump and youthful. Living enzymes found in raw foods are also important for absorbing and incorporating the minerals you eat to build your glowing health and beauty.

COOKED FOODS

Despite the numerous benefits of a diet rich in raw foods, a completely raw diet isn't easy to maintain in colder climates and we naturally crave warming comfort foods on chilly, dark evenings. Diets that are 100% raw can also be quite high in fat, as nuts, seeds, avocados and oils are used abundantly to create dishes. These are certainly healthier choices, but they're still rich in fat and calories and consuming too much of them will lead to weight gain. Raw food also doesn't always agree with those with a weaker digestive system, so lightly steaming food is the better option. But it's really important not to overcook vegetables, as they will lose important water-soluble nutrients like vitamins C and B.

There are some exceptions to the cooked food rule, as certain foods are actually better for us in their cooked form. They also provide the satiety of a heavier and more filling meal. Dinner is the best time to enjoy nourishing cooked foods like quinoa, millet, sweet potato, butternut squash, beans, lentils and lightly steamed veggies. Sweet potatoes and squash can be roasted at high temperatures, yet remain full of essential minerals and nutrients like beta-carotene for brightening your skin. Cooking tomatoes destroys their vitamin C content but increases their levels of lycopene, a powerful antioxidant. After a satisfying evening meal of cooked food, you can relax and allow the digestive process to work, whereas a heavy cooked meal in the middle of the day may compromise your energy levels for the afternoon.

THE BEAUTY OF PROBIOTICS

Literally translated as 'for life', probiotics like *Acidophilus* and *Bifidobacteria* are the beneficial or 'friendly' bacteria normally found in your digestive tract. As the name suggests, they're absolutely essential to life. They help to digest your food properly, they prevent yeast and other 'unfriendly' types of bacteria from overgrowing, they create fatty acids to keep intestinal cells strong and healthy and they produce vitamin K. They're hard-working little micro-organisms!

FRIENDLY GUT BACTERIA

There are *nine* times as many bacteria in your intestinal tract as there are cells in your body, so you want to ensure they're the best type of bacteria. The number and type of bacteria in the gut really matter in beauty, health and disease. Dysbiosis occurs when the 'unfriendly' type begins to have damaging effects on the body because it has overtaken the levels of 'friendly' bacteria. It can also be caused by too much yeast, parasites or viruses. It's an imbalance, and usually your gut bacteria keep a healthy balance of each strain, ensuring that no one strain can dominate. Some of the major reasons for developing dysbiosis include high-protein, high-fat, high-sugar or high-fat diets as well as a low-fibre diet or allergies to certain types of food. It can also be caused by stress, poor digestion, low immune system, infection or antibiotics.

ANTIBIOTICS

Antibiotics are so commonly prescribed now for all types of infections and illnesses that more and more people are developing chronic cases of dysbiosis. Problems associated with it include bloating, weight gain, acne, eczema, psoriasis and fungal nail infections as well as cravings for sugar and alcohol.

Of course, antibiotics are extremely important in certain situations, but the Center for Disease Control describes them as 'grossly over-prescribed'. Antibiotics kill off the bad *and* good bacteria that keep your immune system healthy. Always follow a course of antibiotics with a course of probiotics.

PROBIOTICS FOR HEALTHY SKIN

Regular probiotic use will really help to increase nutrient absorption, smooth out your skin and clear up any pesky skin conditions, reduce bloating and excess weight, improve your hair and nails and even your mood. They're one of the most important tools available for building a more beautiful and radiant you!

I discovered both sauerkraut and coconut water kefir, a probiotic drink, three years ago. Coconut water kefir uses the same kefir grains that are found in milk kefir, but it uses the natural sugars in coconut water to feed the bacteria instead of the sugars in milk. What you get is a slightly sour, fizzy drink that looks like lemonade. Regularly eating sauerkraut and drinking kefir remain the most powerful steps for health and good digestion that I have ever taken. They introduce a host of beneficial enzymes, minerals, vitamins and protein to your body and allow nutrients from the food you eat and digest to be much more effectively absorbed into your bloodstream and body cells to make your skin brighter, clearer and younger looking.

TOP 10 WAYS TO BEAT THE BLOAT

Many of my nutrition clients and friends complain that bloating is an issue for them, with certain foods consistently triggering it. There are a number of reasons for bloating, from food intolerances to poor digestive health and even inadequate water intake, fibre and exercise. If you are switching over to a more plant-based diet rich in fruit and veggies, then it's perfectly normal to feel bloated for the first seven to 10 days while your system adapts to the extra fibre. It's nothing to worry about! If the discomfort and bloating continue, you may want to investigate other possible causes.

Here are my top 10 tips to beat the bloat in just a fortnight or less.

1

FOOD INTOLERANCES

First, isolate and eliminate 'trigger' foods. Gluten in wheat can be particularly difficult for humans to digest and can cause an inflammatory reaction in the intestinal lining, which may lead to a 'leaky' gut and a spectrum of health problems, such as autoimmune diseases. If you suspect that you have an intolerance, try eliminating the food completely for 11 days. On the 12th day, eat as much as you want of that food and then monitor your symptoms over the following two to three days. If the bloating and other discomforts reappear, then it may be best to avoid that food item entirely. The elimination diet is quite a straightforward way of figuring out what food causes problems and many of my clients find it useful. Refined sugar is also a common cause of bloating, as it can encourage unfriendly bacteria and yeast overgrowth in the gut.

2

CHEW YOUR FOOD

Ensure that you're not gulping down your food and swallowing too much air or not chewing it properly. Chew your food well, until it's almost soupy in texture when you swallow it.

3

PROBIOTICS

Take them in capsule form or enjoy them in foods and drinks like sauerkraut, raw apple cider vinegar and coconut water kefir for their huge benefits. A healthy body should have 80–85% friendly bacteria. One of the many reasons I recommend reducing or eliminating animal protein foods is because rotting heavy proteins in our guts create the ideal breeding ground for unhealthy bacteria, creating intestinal toxaemia, accelerated ageing and a whole host of other problems. Meanwhile, good bacteria improve digestion, B vitamin synthesis in the gut and overall energy, enhance nutrient absorption to improve skin and they help to get rid of bloating.

4 TAKE DIGESTIVE ENZYMES

These can really help with digestion. Simply swallow a capsule with some water before a cooked meal and an extra one during the meal if it's particularly heavy or high in fat or animal protein.

5 EAT MORE FIBRE

Consuming plenty of dietary fibre every day is essential for a healthy digestive system and to prevent constipation, a major cause of bloating. Whole fruits, vegetables, gluten-free whole grains, nuts, seeds and legumes are the best sources of fibre.

6 WATER AND EXERCISE

Water is essential to flush out the system and improve peristalsis in the intestine. Aim to drink 2 litres of water per day, and more if you're exercising or during spells of hot weather. Adding a slice of lemon to your water can help enhance the flavour. Regular exercise also helps to reduce bloating, boost the action of the gut and improve lymphatic drainage.

7 EAT FRUIT ON AN EMPTY STOMACH

Avoid eating fruit after a meal because it digests faster than heavier protein and fat-rich foods, causing it to ferment and produce gases that cause bloating.

8 PREBIOTIC FOODS

Certain foods contain prebiotics, which are non-digestible elements that feed and stimulate the action of those all-important probiotics in the gut. These foods include raw bananas, chicory, leek, garlic, onion and Jerusalem artichoke. Try to include one or more of these foods in your diet every day.

9 HERBAL TEAS

Herbal teas are a wonderful replacement for caffeinated drinks and can really help to soothe or stimulate the digestive system. Try peppermint, ginger or fennel and aim to have two to three cups a day.

10 BOOST YOUR ENZYMES

Low hydrochloric acid in your stomach can occur for a number of reasons, and this may lead to bloating and digestive discomfort. Before your main meal, eat a digestion-boosting garden salad or a couple of pieces of raw pineapple or papaya. They contain bromelain and papain respectively, which have proteolytic qualities that can boost the breakdown of protein foods in the stomach. The salad is a 'bitter', which can also boost hydrochloric acid production.

EATING FOR BEAUTY

'ANY FOOD THAT REQUIRES ENHANCING
BY THE USE OF CHEMICAL SUBSTANCES SHOULD
IN NO WAY BE CONSIDERED A FOOD.' *John H. Tobe*

THE PROTEIN MYTH

It's funny – before you become vegan, nobody cares where you get your protein from. But if I tell people now that I don't eat meat, fish, dairy or eggs, their most pressing question is always the protein one. We have been conditioned to believe that the only worthwhile sources of protein are chicken, eggs, meat and fish. I understand that people love their fry-ups, steak dinners, Sunday roasts and scrambled eggs. These meals are often a big part of a person's weekly routine. I'm not suggesting that you give them up *forever*, but for the best beauty and health results, it's important to reduce the amount of animal protein you eat and get creative with the many wonderful sources of nutritious plant protein. It's also a good idea to step away from the status quo and to think beyond the messages that food marketing has bombarded us with for so long.

WHAT IS PROTEIN?

Since its discovery in 1839, protein has been consistently associated with meat. Think of the first food that comes to mind when you say the word *protein*. It's probably beef, or perhaps chicken. Yet there still seems to be a lot of confusion about sources and types of protein. What are good sources? If I give up meat will I become protein deficient? Do I need protein powder and other supplements to build muscles? How do vegetarians get their protein? Do I need to combine different types of plant protein together in the same meal?

It feels like everywhere we look these days, protein is being touted as the wonder nutrient. The message is that we can never get enough protein. Protein is an extremely important part of our diet. It's essential for growth and repair in our bodies and for the production of transport molecules, enzymes, hormones and antibodies. It helps to improve calcium absorption, making it an integral part of bone health, and it helps to improve muscle strength by repairing torn muscle fibres through exercise and everyday wear and tear.

AMINO ACIDS

In total, there are 23 amino acids. Fifteen of these can be made by your body on its own. The remaining eight are known as essential amino acids because they cannot be stored in the body and must be eaten in your diet on a daily basis. A food that contains all eight is called a complete protein. Like beads on a necklace, they form together in various sequences to build the proteins needed for the many everyday biochemical processes in your body. Meat, chicken and eggs are heavily promoted as the only real protein source for building and they go hand in hand for many. But you cannot expect that eating meat will simply turn directly into muscle in your body. We don't just absorb the muscle of an animal into our own muscles. It must first be broken down into amino acids and then they're rebuilt into the protein chains specific to human muscles. These amino acids come from either your diet or your body's own store. If a chronic shortage of amino acids develops, this building ceases to continue and lean muscle may be used to support the body's repair. Your health and beauty will be affected, as lean muscle is so important for a speedy metabolism. Amino acids must be replaced regularly through your food choices. You don't even have to combine different plant protein source into the one meal because your body is cleverly designed to be able to store amino acids and release them as they're needed throughout the day.

Eating some protein with every meal or snack is a great habit to get into as it keeps the levels of amino acids continuously topped up and helps to stabilise blood sugar levels. I add nuts and seeds, nut butters, sprouted lentils, quinoa, tempeh, green veggies and many other great sources of plant-based protein to almost all my meals and I often add a scoop of raw vegan protein powder to post-workout smoothies or use it to make tasty protein balls. It's pretty much impossible to design a diet sufficient in calories and based on whole plant foods that's deficient in any of the amino acids. The one exception could be a diet based purely on fruit.

Hemp seeds are one of my favourite complete plant proteins to add to salads, soups and smoothies. Just 3 tablespoons of hemp seeds provide 10 grams of protein to help you feel full and keep blood sugar levels steady.

PLANT PROTEIN BOOSTS BEAUTY

There are numerous sources of plant-based amino acids built into a nutrient-rich package to shed extra pounds, bring out your beauty and make you glow with health. When I first switched over to a vegan diet, I was amazed at the variety of foods available. Gone were the tasteless egg whites, processed protein powders and fat-free cottage cheese, and in their place I began eating an abundance of vibrant plant foods.

GREENS

Green vegetables come in a nutritionally perfect assortment of fibre, phytonutrients, minerals, vitamins, antioxidants and essential fatty acids. Calorie for calorie, leafy greens are the most nutritious type of food to eat.

NUTS AND SEEDS

Nuts, seeds and nut and seed butters are packed with protein and essential fats for health and beauty. Eaten raw, almonds, walnuts, chia seeds, pumpkin seeds and many others are a superb source of plant protein. However, they are a dense food, so about a handful a day is a good amount to aim for, or a little more if you're extremely active or trying to gain weight.

Our shops and supermarkets are full of roasted and salted nuts and seeds, but they will benefit your health most when eaten in their natural state.* Roasting them can destroy their amino acids and healthy fatty acids, plus they're often cooked in unhealthy vegetable oils.

BEANS AND LEGUMES

All varieties of beans and legumes are another excellent source of inexpensive plant protein and are a staple in my diet. I always have a sprouting jar in my kitchen filled with lentils, chickpeas, broccoli seeds, alfalfa and adzuki beans. Once I have soaked them for a few hours to stimulate germination, they only take a couple of days to fully sprout. It's like having my own greenhouse on speed on my windowsill! But in cooler months, cooked beans and legumes add a satisfying warmth and density to the diet without having to worry about gaining 'hibernation weight' over the winter, because beans are naturally low in fat and high in fibre. They're also high in minerals like iron, calcium and magnesium, plus vitamins and phytonutrients to fight against ageing.

It's better to avoid canned foods altogether due to the various chemicals in them, so I advise buying dried beans in bulk and soaking and cooking them yourself. To cook dried beans, first soak the beans in a large bowl of water overnight, ensuring they are completely submerged in the water. The next day, drain the beans and transfer them to a large saucepan. Cover them with double their volume of water and bring them to a boil for 5 minutes. Cover partly with a lid, reduce the heat and simmer for approximately 1 hour, until the beans are cooked through and tender. Add more water if necessary to keep the beans submerged while they're cooking. Drain well and use as required in the recipe.

PROTEIN POWDERS

I used to drink the popular whey-based protein shakes every day, and their slick marketing promised to transform me into a sleek, ripped athlete. It didn't happen! Unfortunately, protein powders are usually highly processed, heat treated and full of preservatives. You can get all the amino acids you need from real food. But if you're a gym-goer and you feel that you need an extra boost after a weights workout, then I recommend a good-quality hemp protein powder or the Sunwarrior raw vegan protein powder. After a tough gym session, I usually pop a scoop or two of Sunwarrior protein powder into a smoothie with spinach, blueberries and unsweetened almond milk to boost my muscle recovery.

HIGH-PROTEIN DIETS: THE UGLY TRUTH

Over the past few decades, high-protein, low-carb diets have surged in popularity, yet based on the scientific research that is now emerging, the potential health risks are huge. I've tried high-protein diets in the past, drawn in by the hype, and they left me tired, lethargic, foggy-headed and grumpy, with bad breath and no energy to exercise. Yes, they can help to reduce a bit of bloating and you may lose a few pounds of water weight, but that shoots straight back on the moment you eat a regular meal.

High-protein diets based on animal foods can often lack the fibre, phytochemicals and other nutrients you need for optimal health and beauty. Apart from the many health dangers, the fact is that high-protein diets will cause you to age faster because they're based on foods devoid of fibre and low in the nutrients and antioxidants needed to mop up the free radicals circulating in your system. A surplus of animal protein foods will not boost your beauty or give you glowing skin and shiny hair. Instead, they leave an acidic residue in your blood after digestion, which challenges your body to balance itself with alkaline minerals.

CHOOSE ANIMAL PROTEIN WISELY

The mentality of eating all the animal protein you can in a meal will not improve your beauty or health in the long term. While you don't need to eat meat for nutrition, there are plenty of reasons why you might still want to include animal-based foods in your diet. My advice is to simply choose wisely and enjoy it in moderation, balanced out with plenty of fresh, whole plant foods. Eating a serving of meat, poultry, fish or eggs a maximum of two to three times a week is enough, and try to eat them for your evening meal so your body can spend time digesting. Buy organic, free-range, grass-fed meat that is free from hormones. A local farmer or trusted family butcher is often the best option, and it helps to know that the animals are treated as humanely as possible. If you do choose to eat meat, then small quantities of very good-quality animal protein are better than large amounts of lesser-quality meat.

Oily fish is a better option than meat as it's easier to digest and comes with the added benefits of essential omega-3 oils. But I still recommend that you limit fish and seafood to once or twice a week. Like other animal protein foods, it digests to leave an acidic residue. Fish is also known to be a polluted food and is often contaminated with mercury, dioxin and PCBs. The best choice is wild salmon for its fatty acids, but don't confuse this with Atlantic salmon, which is farmed. Farmed fish can also be fed various dyes to give them that characteristic pink salmon colour, which you definitely don't want in your precious body!

BEAUTIFUL CARBOHYDRATES

Who doesn't crave an enormous feed of bread, pasta, spaghetti, rice or mashed potatoes when the evenings get chilly and dark? Carbohydrates are the ultimate comfort food. They create a warm, full belly and sleepy contentment. We're so accustomed to seeing 'low-carb', 'carb-free' and 'sugar-free' written on food packaging, and many popular diets have demonised carbs and made carb-counting popular. But carbs deserve a second chance. They're not all that bad!

The best carbs you can eat for beautiful skin and a lean body are the unprocessed, complex type. They contain plenty of fibre, which means that they take longer for your system to digest, release their glucose slowly into your bloodstream and keep you satiated for a much longer period of time. They will also boost your beauty and health the most and help you to maintain your ideal weight.

Starchy vegetables are incredibly good for your beauty and health. They're a great addition to a meal as they're so filling and rich in fibre, vitamins and minerals. The very best types include sweet potato, all types of squash and pumpkin.

Gluten-free grains are another wonderful and satisfying way to add high-quality carbs to your diet. The best choices are quinoa, millet, amaranth and buckwheat, as they're easy to digest and leave an alkaline residue in your blood. Brown, black and wild rice are also great choices and go well with veggie curries and stews and can even be added to soups to make them more filling. Most of these grains can be found in good supermarkets and they tend to be pretty inexpensive, making them a nutritious option for those watching the pennies. I often make a big batch of quinoa with veggies, which can be stored in an airtight container in the fridge for a few days. Compared to white rice or refined wheat-based carbs like pasta, bread and couscous, these grains are of far superior quality and will add good nutrition, fibre and density to your diet without affecting blood sugar levels or causing bloating and weight gain.

Beans, peas and lentils are another ideal type of starch. They also just so happen to be high in fibre, protein and essential minerals like iron and calcium. All varieties of beans, lentils and peas should feature in your diet regularly. They help you to feel full and satisfied and are incredibly versatile.

REFINED CARBOHYDRATES

Avoid refined carbohydrates as much as possible. These include white flour, breads, pastas, pastries, white rice, crisps, many breakfast cereals and most packaged foods, such as biscuits, cakes, crackers and baked treats. The refinement process used to produce these foods removes the bran and germ of the grain, which depletes it of fibre and many of its vitamins, minerals and other nutrients. Other refined sugars to avoid include sucrose, lactose, fruit juice concentrates and glucose-fructose corn syrup. Drinking alcohol also places heavy stress on blood sugar control in the body and can cause levels to fluctuate.

Refined sugar is one of the most damaging foods you can eat, as it creates extreme fluctuations in energy, intense cravings for another sugar hit and emotions including anxiety, depression, anger and negativity. Your brain is the first to suffer from low blood sugar levels, as it depends on glucose as its main source of energy. Simple carbs offer a quick burst of energy to the body, but this can also cause your blood sugar to quickly rise, as it triggers the pancreas to release insulin, which stores the excess glucose as fat. You'll often experience a crash a few hours later, creating a cycle of cravings and addiction.

The problems begin when carbohydrates are refined, as they've had their fibre and many of their vitamins, minerals and other nutrients removed, and the rate that they get absorbed into your blood quickly increases. This causes an emotional and physical roller coaster of sugar highs and lows. Forcing the pancreas to consistently produce insulin may eventually lead to insulin resistance, which has been associated in numerous clinical trials with obesity and illness. We donate plenty of our own energy to digesting these foods, but as they're so devoid of nutrients, they rob us of valuable energy and deplete our body of its vital beauty nutrients, including magnesium, vitamin C needed for plump skin and B vitamins for energy production and weight loss.

The very best way to stabilise blood sugar levels to feel calm, balanced and satisfied throughout the day is by eating a diet high in fibre and complex carbs. If you battle with your weight, constantly snack on sugary treats and suffer from energy highs and lows, then it's an addictive cycle that must be broken. Refined sugar is the worst type of food you can eat if you're trying to lose body fat and improve your energy levels.

SUGAR ADDICTION

I was a sugar addict in my teens and early twenties. I ate foods that I thought were healthy because they were labelled 'low-fat' or 'fat-free', but they were actually packed full of refined sugar. Diet yoghurts, cereal bars, sweetened instant coffee, baked beans and packet soups all featured in my diet. Energy drinks made their way in during stressful university exam times too. I used to crave jelly sweets, sugary ice pops and chocolate and needed to get my fix regularly. On those frequent trips to the student bar, I always ordered a brightly coloured, sickly sweet blue or pink alcopop. So I know exactly what it's like to be in the grasp of a sugar addiction. Sometimes we're not even truly aware of it or live in denial of it. But looking back, I really struggled with my fluctuating energy levels, emotions and skin breakouts. I was always sporty and played netball and

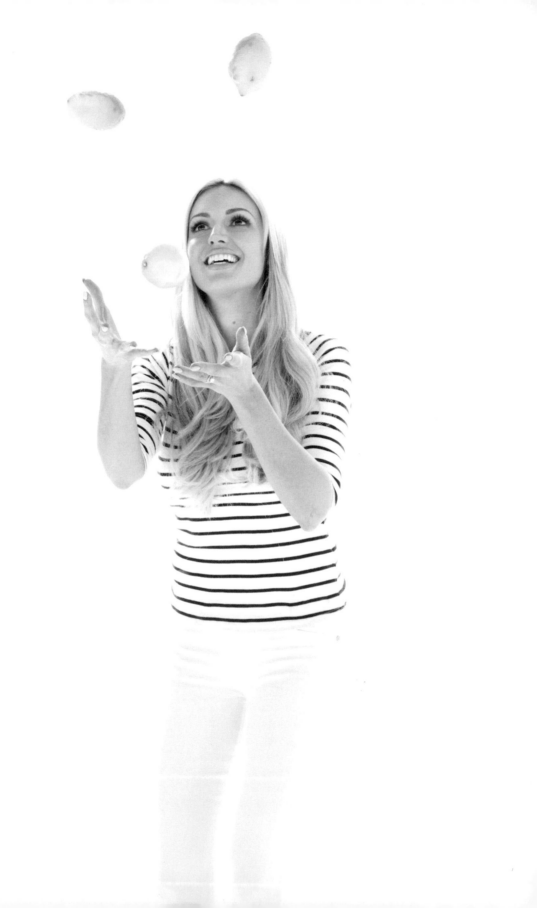

went to the gym and Pilates classes regularly, so I was lucky that my weight stayed pretty stable. But I often battled colds, flu, sniffles and niggling health problems linked to a low immune system, because sugar is known to damage our special immune system cells and leave us more vulnerable to illness.

When I decided to quit sugar completely overnight, I struggled at the beginning. Our taste buds renew themselves every 10 days, so we can change the way we taste foods quite quickly. Three weeks is generally a good length of time to aim for to drop a habit and get rid of cravings. Now, refined sugar tastes sickeningly sweet to me and I can immediately tell if it's been snuck into my food. Fruit is sweet enough for me now, and if I'm really craving a sweet treat, I'll make a healthy dessert or whizz up a smoothie.

REFINED SUGAR AND PREMATURE AGEING

Sugar doesn't just wreak havoc on your weight, emotions and health; it's also one of the worst foods to eat if you want clear, young-looking skin. It's a sly villain, tempting you with its taste and causing chaos to your body and beauty.

According to dermatologist and nutritionist Dr Nicholas Perricone, sugar is as bad for your skin as it is for your waistline. When your body breaks down carbs to glucose during digestion, your pancreas releases insulin to deal with the increase in blood sugar levels. But the insulin spike you get when you eat processed or sugary foods is described by Perricone as 'a burst of inflammation throughout the body', which damages your connective tissues too. This inflammation creates enzymes that break down the important proteins respon-sible for your skin's structure and firmness, called collagen and elastin. Over time, this creates crow's feet, fine lines and sagging skin, especially around the jowls.
But sugar also speeds up the rate at which

your skin ages through a process called glycation. Digested sugar attaches itself to your skin's collagen and forms advanced glycation end products, which is appro-priately shortened to AGEs. These cause the important protein fibres in your skin to become hard and stiff instead of soft, plump and supple. This shows up on your skin as lines and wrinkles, sagging and dullness. Furthermore, having AGEs in your skin also makes your complexion far more susceptible to toxins in cigarette smoke and UV damage, particularly as you get older. Glycation can also worsen acne and rosacea. Unfortu-nately, the signs of damage from glycation tend to show themselves from about the age of 30: an accumulation of hormonal changes, sun damage, oxidative stress from the environment and the creation of AGEs from our diet. In our childhood, teens and twenties, our body is much better able to repair any damage and produce plenty of collagen. As we get older, toxic damage builds up and our ability to repair decreases.

Even healthy foods like fruit, veggies and certain grains turn to glucose when digested, though in a much less damaging way, plus they contain antioxidants and other nutrients to dampen down inflammation and mop up toxins. Also, there's no way you could cut out all carbs because glucose is so integral to all of your metabolic processes. It keeps us *alive*! For most healthy individuals with nothing wrong with their glucose levels, the process of glycation is a normal part of life and happens at a gradual rate. But your diet and lifestyle choices can really speed up the ageing process. Glycation can't be halted completely, but it can be slowed down. A high-sugar diet plus smoking and not taking care of your skin in the sun are three of the main factors in ageing.

GLUCOSE-FRUCTOSE SYRUP

High-fructose corn syrup is one of the very worst types of sugar for ageing us quickly. In the US it's called high-fructose corn syrup, but in Ireland and the UK it's known as glucose-fructose syrup. It's a cheap and refined type of sweetener made from corn and is often found in fizzy drinks, cereals, biscuits and other sweet baked snacks. It contains glucose and a very high level of fructose, which actually gets changed to and stored as fat even more quickly than glucose.

Glucose-fructose syrup hits your liver straight away and has been linked to the development of fatty liver disease, even in those who don't drink alcohol. Keep it away from your delicate body, as refined sugar and starch will impede weight loss and damage your looks. You don't need it in your life and the cycle of sugar addiction *can* be broken! To preserve your skin and keep it looking young for as long as possible, I strongly advise you to either totally eliminate sugar or dramatically reduce it from your diet. This means checking packaging, as it can sneak into many savoury foods as well as the more obvious sweet foods, such as pasta sauces, soups, chutneys, bread, cream cheese, crackers, dips, dressings, jam, yoghurts, cereals, juices and junk foods. I used to be addicted to tomato ketchup and sweet chilli sauce and put them on everything. I sadly waved goodbye to them when I cut out sugar and now they taste unbearably sweet to me.

SAFE SWEETENERS

Humans are naturally drawn to sweet tastes, and it's absolutely fine to enjoy sweet treats *in moderation*. My favourite sweetener to use is stevia, which I buy as a liquid and as a powder. It's sold in most health food shops and some supermarkets, but take care that you don't buy the version of stevia mixed into Splenda, as that's a chemical sweetener to avoid. I also like to use xylitol, which is a natural sugar alcohol. Organic dried and fresh fruit make excellent sugar substitutes for desserts too. Try blending together summer berries with vanilla seeds for a healthy coulis. Other safe sweeteners include honey, which isn't vegan but can be used in moderation. Make sure it's local, raw, organic honey for the most benefits. High-quality, organic maple syrup is another sweetener I like to use in occasional sweet treats, as it has such a rich flavour. Again, only a small amount is ever needed, and although it's not raw because it has to be heat treated, it's still less processed than agave. Blackstrap molasses is rich in iron, calcium, copper and magnesium and works well in baking. Coconut sugar and coconut blossom nectar are also good choices.

AVOID AGAVE

Agave has been marketed as a healthy, all-natural sweetener with a low glycaemic index, but it has actually been highly processed before it reaches your desserts and pancakes. However, the major problem with agave is that is contains up to 90% fructose, which is far more than glucose-fructose syrup and is bad for your weight, health and complexion. Agave is simply not worth the health risks and it won't support your beauty and body goals.

SAY GOODBYE TO GLUTEN

'Gluten-free' is increasingly used to sell various food products, but is it all a bit of a fad and an excuse to avoid carbs? And what exactly is gluten anyway? Gluten is the protein found in wheat, barley and rye, but oats can contain it if they have been cross-contaminated by gluten grains in transport and storage. It's what makes bread chewy and delicious, and it's also found in beer, soy sauce, pasta, bagels, sauces, pizza, crackers, cake, soups, ice cream, some veggie burgers, biscuits, sausages, breakfast cereals and many other processed foods.

Ever since dietary guidelines called for us to lower our intake of fat a few decades ago, the Western world has become fatter and sicker than ever before. Refined sugar is definitely a culprit, but modern wheat has been genetically altered from the staple food of our ancestors to enable the manufacturers of processed food to get the greatest yield for the lowest cost.

GLUTEN SENSITIVITY

You may have heard of the link between coeliac disease and gluten, but wheat can actually be responsible for more than just coeliac disease. A lesser-known set of serious side effects of gluten consumption is referred to under the umbrella term 'non-coeliac gluten sensitivity'. This is a sensitivity to gluten that does not show up as intestinal issues, but according to research it can lead to health conditions like arthritis, depression, eczema and psoriasis. Persistent acne and weight gain are two other major symptoms associated with non-coeliac gluten sensitivity. Gluten can trigger inflammation in the body, which often manifests in our skin as acne. It's accompanied by a disruption in friendly gut bacteria and greater intestinal permeability. Wheat is not a beauty-boosting food and it won't help you to achieve your utmost health potential.

If you find it impossible to clear up your skin or lose those few extra stubborn pounds no matter what you do, it's time to look at the role of gluten in your diet. Moving to a gluten-free diet will enable more fruits, veggies, nuts, seeds, avocados and gluten-free whole grains to be a part of your diet, which will also help to heal your skin.

There are so many nutrient-rich foods available to replace wheat products, like quinoa, millet, buckwheat, brown rice and amaranth. There's also a multitude of flours available to replace regular flour in baking, including chickpea, brown rice, coconut, buckwheat, almond and quinoa flours. There are plenty of gluten-free products on the shelves now and they can be so helpful if you are transitioning away from gluten, but read the ingredients list carefully and avoid anything overly processed.

THE F WORD

Fat. It's a dirty word, right? Nobody wants to be called the F word, and low-fat or even fat-free foods have become a staple for the figure-conscious amongst us. Yet fat is essential to life itself. Fat helps to keep your joints supple and your skin soft and youthful, and polyunsaturated fats are essential components of nerve cells and cell membranes.

Your liver can synthesise enough cholesterol to carry out its important functions in the body, but essential fatty acids (EFAs) are needed for optimal health and cannot be made in the body. Therefore, it's crucial to include the right balance of EFAs in your daily diet from specific foods. These are omega-3, omega-6 and omega-9 fats. People generally eat too many omega-6 and 9 fats in animal-based foods, vegetable oils and margarine, but many are borderline deficient in omega-3 fats. A large proportion of clients I've seen and treated have shown classic symptoms of an omega-3 fat deficiency.

One of the major health benefits of EFAs is their powerful ability to reduce inflammation in the body, too much of which can lead to skin problems and poor health. Good plant-based food sources include flaxseeds, hemp seeds, chia seeds, raw walnuts, leafy green vegetables, avocado and micro-algae, such as chlorella and spirulina. In fact, micro-algae is the finest source of these essential nutrients because the oil has the optimum balance of DHA to EPA. Your body puts it directly to work without the multi-step conversion processes of other forms of omega-3.

It's a great idea to include a serving of one of these foods in your diet each day. It's an added beauty incentive that your skin is one of the first places you will really notice an improvement in when you start adding more healthy fats to your diet. Mine became softer, smoother and less prone to dryness, especially during the winter months.

BAD FATS

Unfortunately, our modern diet tends to be based on too much of the wrong type of fat. Fat is the most concentrated form of energy available to us, but we only need small amounts of essential fat. As an adult, about one-third of our daily calories should come from fat. For optimal health, beauty and your ideal weight, it's important to reduce your intake of saturated fats, cholesterol and trans fatty acids. Trans fatty acids, found in most processed foods like commercial cakes, biscuits and margarine, have been associated with ill health. Saturated fats and cholesterol are found primarily in animal products such as meat, cheese, chocolate, ice cream and milk. It's the marbling you can see in meats like beef and pork. We do need some saturated fat to allow our liver to make cholesterol, but too much can raise blood LDL cholesterol. The easiest way to reduce levels of saturated fat and cholesterol is to eat less animal foods and more low-fat, high-fibre plant foods, such as fruit, vegetables, legumes and gluten-free grains.

VEGETABLE OILS

It can be all too easy to overeat oils because they lack the fibre to tell us when we're feeling full and are packed with calories, as they're 100% fat. I avoid oils almost completely and rarely cook with them at home, because eating the whole source of the food is so much more beneficial. For example, I eat whole olives rather than olive oil. Even the cold-pressed extra virgin olive oil drizzled on your salad will cover the nutrients in a coat of fat and slow down the rate that they're absorbed at. Yes, we need fat to help the absorption of various vitamins, but a handful of nuts and seeds or a few slices of creamy avocado will do that job perfectly.

COCONUT OIL

Coconut oil is a great fat to cook with because it has a high smoke point and doesn't produce toxic compounds when heated. But other types of cooking oils are amongst the most ageing, fattening and unhealthy oils you can consume. Think of the heated cooking oils used to fry chips, burgers and other fried foods. Eating this type of fat too often can lead to weight gain, premature ageing, acne and other skin complaints as well as placing a strain on your liver and digestive system. While coconut oil is still pure fat and needs to be eaten in moderation because it will fatten you up if you enjoy too much too often, it's an excellent addition to desserts, stir-fries and roast veggies. It's an oil that's easy to digest and is used as a source of quick, clean energy. Although it contains up to 90% saturated fat, coconut oil is free from cholesterol and trans fats. Over half of the fatty acids in coconut oil is lauric acid, which has been shown to support thyroid health, and boost metabolism as a result, because the thyroid controls metabolism. Apart from a little cooked coconut oil, always aim to eat fats in their raw, natural and unprocessed state. Your skin, body and brain will really thank you for it.

DAIRY

I've already mentioned the visit I made to a dietician soon after I switched to a fully vegetarian diet in my late teens. After just one week of consuming three servings of dairy products a day, as she had recommended, my skin developed an acne breakout and my abdomen was uncomfortably bloated. I immediately cut cow's milk products from my diet and have avoided them ever since. The acne and bloating disappeared as quickly as they had started. Personally, it's been one of the most important steps I have taken for preventing problem skin and spotty breakouts.

Throughout my years of clinical training in college and the subsequent work I've done with clients, dairy has consistently emerged as a problematic type of food for some people. This was confirmed by the food intolerance blood tests that many of my clients chose to take.

I recommended that these clients seek out calcium-rich dairy alternatives in place of dairy products and advised them on the best plant-based sources of calcium. All reported health improvements within the first four weeks, most notably clearer skin and weight loss. It's useful for those trying to lose weight to note that a glass of unsweetened Alpro almond milk contains just 32.5 calories, compared to 100 calories in a 250ml glass of slimline cow's milk.

As you know, nature intended cow's milk to feed a newborn calf in its early stages of life. Humans are the only species on earth that drinks the milk of another mammal and continues to do so as adults. However, scientists at the prestigious US Harvard School of Public Health have announced that milk is not the best source of calcium for healthy bones, citing widespread lactose intolerance and a high saturated fat content, among other things, as particularly relevant reasons to seek out calcium from plant-based sources:

'There is little if any evidence that high dairy intakes protect against osteoporosis, and there is considerable evidence that too-high intakes can be harmful. Plus, dairy products can be high in saturated fat as well as retinol (vitamin A), which at high levels can paradoxically weaken bones.'

Yet this is a staple food found in every grocery shop, sold to all of us from school-going age as a great food for humans. In a paper published in the *Journal of the American Medical Association Pediatrics*, Harvard paediatrics professor David Ludwig, MD, PhD, writes:

'Humans have no nutritional requirement for animal milk, an evolutionarily recent addition to the diet. Anatomically, modern humans presumably achieved adequate nutrition for millennia before domestication of dairy animals, and many populations throughout the world today consume little or no milk for biological reasons (lactase deficiency), lack of availability or cultural preferences. Adequate dietary calcium for bone health ... can be obtained from many other sources. Throughout the world, bone fracture rates tend to be lower in countries that do not consume milk compared to those that do.'

There are arguments for the inclusion of dairy as a necessary and important part of our diets, and many make valid points, such as the level of calcium that can be found in dairy products. However, this was not my experience, or that of a number of my clients over the years, so I look to other foods to satisfy my calcium intake.

DAIRY AND YOUR SKIN

Removing dairy from my diet worked wonders for clearing up my own complexion, and I've seen huge improvements in clients who come to me with acne and other inflammatory skin conditions. Scientific studies have confirmed an association between acne and drinking milk, with a 2008 study published in the *Journal of the American Academy of Dermatology* concluding that skimmed milk contains hormones in large enough quantities to affect our own hormones and lead to acne.

My advice to anyone who suffers from acne is to avoid dairy for three to four weeks to see if that makes any difference. If it does, then getting used to dairy alternatives and high-calcium, plant-based foods is the best option for encouraging clear, inflammation-free skin.

YOGHURT

I know so many health-conscious people who have given up milk and cheese but continue to eat yoghurt. Yoghurt is heavily promoted as the perfect snack for children and fitness fans, but it's no different to milk. Yoghurt is advertised as being a great source of friendly probiotic bacteria, but many of these products are full of refined sugar, which actually feeds the *unhealthy* gut bacteria and encourages it to flourish. Sauerkraut, dairy-free kefir and probiotic capsules as well as a high-fibre, whole foods diet are all far better ways to look after your gut flora.

WHAT'S THE ALTERNATIVE?

Dairy products may be promoted as the best source of calcium for growing and maintaining bone mass, and it's true that they do contain plenty of calcium. But plant sources of the mineral generally contain magnesium, potassium, folic acid, boron and vitamins C and K, which are all essential for laying down bone. Both vitamin D and magnesium are important for the proper absorption of calcium. Dairy products are not a very good source of magnesium, and consuming too much will actually block magnesium from being properly absorbed.

Calcium-fortified plant milks are widely available in shops, supermarkets, hotels and restaurants these days, so finding a dairy alternative that suits your taste and budget shouldn't be a problem. When I removed dairy from my diet, I lost weight, my energy and fitness improved and I felt better than ever before.

THINK GREEN AND LEAN

The best foods to eat for both calcium and magnesium in easily absorbed forms are dark green leafy veggies like spinach, kale, broccoli, Brussels sprouts, cabbage, watercress and turnip greens. Other good food sources include almonds, asparagus, beans and legumes, sesame seeds and tahini, walnuts, Brazil nuts and both fresh and dried figs.

Leafy green veggies, green peas and oats are all superb sources of vitamin K1, which dramatically slows down bone loss. These foods also contain high amounts of calcium and the trace mineral boron to further protect bones. Fruit and vegetables are the best dietary source of boron, and a diet deficient in them may also be low in boron.

VEGETABLES: THE ULTIMATE BEAUTY FOOD

Raw green vegetables are the most important type of food that you need to eat in order to become as bright-eyed, glowing, beautiful, lean and healthy as you possibly can. It couldn't be easier! There's no magic pill, potion or lotion in the world that will do what abundant greens can do for your complexion. For the alkalising minerals, amino acids and living enzymes that you need for your health, raw greens are the most nutrient-rich of all foods. Their green pigment, chlorophyll, shares the same molecular structure as the haemoglobin in your own blood, making it a powerful tool in cleansing and reinvigorating your blood and body cells. I eat greens with every meal to get the most benefit. Building meals around big salads or ordering a salad, steamed broccoli or spinach on the side are great ways to get your greens in.

Almost all types of vegetables leave an alkaline residue when they are digested, which makes them especially good for your beauty and health. Eating fresh, organic produce is ideal, of course, but frozen vegetables can be rich in nutrients too if fresh isn't as easily available. It's best to avoid canned vegetables altogether, as they can be high in salt, preservatives and other toxic chemicals.

Eating and drinking a lot of raw alkaline veggies will do wonders for your detoxification and healing, but in cooler climates, roasted and steamed vegetables are also a super option. Lightly steaming or stir-frying broccoli, Brussels sprouts, green beans, bok choy and asparagus can make them easier to digest while still keeping some of their vitamins and living enzymes intact. Roasting Portobello mushrooms, tomatoes, peppers, onions and carrots can be a delicious and satisfying component to an evening meal. Starch-based veggies like squash, pumpkin, parsnips, turnips and sweet potato need to be cooked well to be at their most digestible and health-promoting, as they're bursting with fibre, minerals and beta-carotene for glowing skin.

EAT THE RAINBOW

You may be familiar with the catchphrase 'eat the rainbow', and not just from Skittles ads! It's to remind us to eat a selection of colourful vegetables every day to benefit from their wide array of phytonutrients, minerals, enzymes and vitamins. The colour of your food can tell you a lot about its levels of nutrients and antioxidants. Orange and yellow fruits and veggies are full of vitamins A and C, while greens are rich in vitamins B, E and K and purple plants are packed with vitamins C and K. But it's really the spectrum of protective phytochemicals found in different colours that matters for your skin, hair and health. For the very best range of beauty benefits, you must add a variety of colourful plant foods to your daily diet.

BEAUTIFUL FRUIT

Fruit is my favourite food, especially the sweet, juicy, tropical types, plus grapes and berries of every variety. They are nature's candy in a nutritionally perfect package. Fruit also happens to be the most beautifying type of food you can eat, thanks to its rich content of water, fibre, vitamins, minerals and antioxidants. The high levels of polyphenolic flavonoids, anthocyanins and vitamin C in various types of fruit are the main reasons why they help to keep your skin healthy and plump, improve your immune system and protect you from illness. Fruit is also the fastest type of food to digest, breaking down to leave an alkaline residue and supplying you with clean-burning, instant energy.

BERRIES

Berries rank the highest of all fruits for their antioxidant concentration. Just one cup of berries provides all the antioxidants you need in a day to prevent disease and slow down the ageing process. Blueberries, blackberries and cranberries come out on top, followed closely by apples, mangos, melons and peaches. They're also easy to find in almost all supermarkets, though some are more seasonal than others. Purple, blue, red and orange fruits offer significant beauty benefits – sweet cherries, raspberries, strawberries, black plums and red grapes all contain a staggering volume of antioxidants, vitamins and flavonoids such as catechin, quercetin and anthocyanidin. These are some of nature's most beautifying compounds, deliciously presented as juicy, sweet, life-enhancing goodness.

EAT FRUIT RAW

Fruit is brimming with living enzymes and delicate vitamins, so it's best enjoyed in its natural, raw state, as heating can destroy much of the goodness. Dried fruit like prunes, dates, figs and dried cranberries also pack an impressive antioxidant punch, but because they're lower in water and higher in more concentrated sugar, they're best enjoyed sparingly and work well in the occasional dessert or sweet treat. Always try to buy organic dried fruit, free from sulphites and other preservatives, added sugar and oil.

HAPPY BANANAS

Ripe bananas are a true feel-good beauty food. They're high in vitamin B6, which is needed to produce the 'happy hormone', serotonin, and the 'sleep hormone', melatonin, so eating bananas regularly can improve your mood, reduce cravings for sugar and carbs and lead to a better night's sleep. They also make a brilliant snack when you're on the go, as they're high in fibre, energy and nutrients to keep you feeling satisfied and less likely to reach for sugary or fatty snacks.

FRUIT AND BLOATING

Although fruit is relatively low in calories and almost fat free, some people may experience bloating and water retention after eating it. I used to have this problem when I began transitioning from a high-protein, low-carb diet to a whole foods, plant-based diet. I had previously restricted my fruit intake to just a handful of blueberries a day, as I worried that any more than that would be too much sugar. So when I began adding more sweet fruit to smoothies and eating it as a snack, I did suffer from bloating. But when I began focusing on my digestive system's health, my ability to digest fruit improved hugely.

You need plenty of friendly gut bacteria to efficiently break down the simple sugars in fruit. If you have been regularly prescribed antibiotics, suffer from thrush or recurrent fungal infections or have been eating a diet high in animal protein, fat or processed food, then you may have an imbalance in the beneficial gut bacteria that you need to properly digest, absorb and assimilate fruit. You will likely experience bloating and discomfort from sweeter fruits. I strongly recommend that you focus on healing your digestive system and eat low-sugar blueberries and citrus fruits rather than sweet fruits for six to eight weeks.

SMOOTHIES AND JUICES

Would you like to have clear skin, shiny hair, strong nails and a lean, supple body without investing a small fortune in beauty treatments? Of course you would! Smoothies are one of the most beautifying of all categories of food and drinks. They should be the foundation of your diet, and they're a major part of the *Eat Yourself Beautiful* programme and lifestyle.

Four years ago, I began drinking a green smoothie every morning and it made a noticeable difference to my skin, hair, nails and body shape. I felt leaner and fitter, my skin began to glow and my hair grew stronger and shinier. The secret to smoothies is that they enable you to consume a large quantity of nutrition in one go and in the way that nature intended, with all the fibre, juice and nutrients intact. I have included all my favourite smoothie recipes for you to choose from in the recipe section. Investing in a sturdy blender will really help you to keep on track with your healthy diet.

THE GREEN GODDESS SMOOTHIE

I have nicknamed my favourite green smoothie blend 'the green goddess' because of its incredible power to make you feel strong, energetic, beautiful and deeply nourished.

I'm regularly asked if it's healthy to use fruit in smoothies and juices because of their sugar content, but I always aim to make my fruit and veggie smoothies with 70–80%

greens and 20–30% fruit. If you're new to blending, then you may prefer to use a little more fruit and a few drops of liquid stevia also help to sweeten it. But my favourite combination of baby spinach with cucumber, banana, pineapple, blueberries, mint, ginger and lime is delicious when served ice cold and you won't even taste the greens, I promise! The fruit hides any 'green' flavour, and as it's blended in its whole form rather than juiced, all the fibre remains intact. This makes it much healthier than fruit juice and prevents a blood sugar spike.

Compared to juices, a smoothie keeps you feeling full and more satisfied. I recommend drinking a green goddess smoothie first thing in the morning after a glass of warm water with lemon. The recipe is on page 218.

JUICING

Juicing is a brilliant way to incorporate a wealth of goodness into your diet. Pure green juice is my top choice, as it's jam-packed with chlorophyll for cleansed blood and glowing skin, oxygen to regenerate your blood and cells, and living enzymes, vitamins, minerals and antioxidants to restore your body, remove waste products and alkalise the blood. The major difference between a juice and a smoothie is that there is almost no fibre in juice. This means that the goodness of the juice gets absorbed into your bloodstream much more quickly. However, it can also be so cleansing to your body that if you have a less balanced system, you may experience more severe detox symptoms, including headache, chills and joint and muscle aches and pains.

Green juice is natural liquid vitality, delivered straight to your cells. It has numerous alkalising benefits, but it doesn't keep you full in the same way that a smoothie will due to the lack of fibre. I drink green juice quite regularly, but the green goddess smoothie on page 218 is my daily staple as it satiates me for much longer and makes it a

useful way to manage body weight.

Green juice can be prepared in large batches and frozen ahead of time, as the nutrients remain intact in the freezer. When buying green juice, always make sure that it's raw, cold pressed and organic if possible. Unfortunately, most commercial vegetable juices are heat treated, which destroys the valuable vitamins and denatures the living enzymes. Dead, denatured food will not build beautiful, vibrant cells. Some of the best veggies to juice include kale, celery, cucumber, beetroot, carrot, parsley, spinach, watercress and wheatgrass. Avocado and banana are best puréed and then added into the juice afterwards. Fruit juice is the most cleansing of all, but I recommend minimising the amount of fruit juice you drink because it hits the bloodstream too quickly and will cause your insulin levels to spike. It's best to enjoy fruit in its whole form or in smoothies, with the fibre intact, and most of the juice you drink should be green. For an extra immune system boost, try adding a clove of raw garlic if you're feeling brave! Always wash fruit and vegetables thoroughly before juicing, remove tough skins, apple cores and pips, and if you are using non-organic produce, scrub it well to remove waxes and pesticides.

WATER

Water is an essential nutrient. It's fundamental to all bodily functions because our body is two-thirds water. It helps to convey nutrients and waste into and out of cells and is needed for water-soluble vitamins like B and C to be used properly.

Each day, we lose around six to 10 glasses of water through our kidneys, skin, lungs and faeces, which is why it's so important to replace this water by drinking at least eight glasses a day, or more in the heat or if you're exercising. I've watched friends, family and

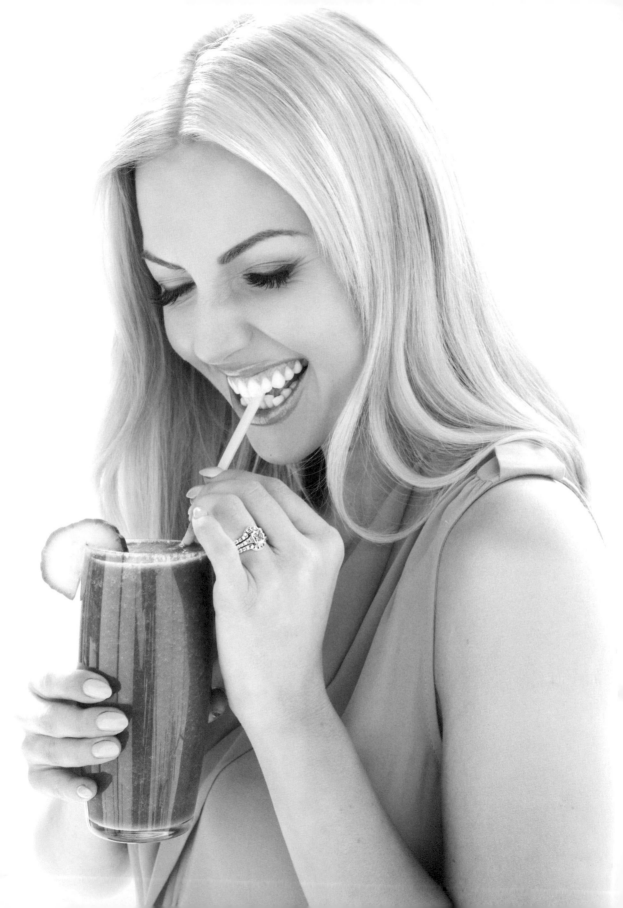

clients transform their skin and health and even lose weight simply by upping their water intake. Did you know that when we're dehydrated, our brains can often interpret it as hunger? So we reach for a quick snack when we should just take a moment to drink a glass of water.

VITAMINS, MINERALS AND SUPPLEMENTS

Just like protein, carbohydrates, fats, water and living enzymes, vitamins and minerals are crucial for keeping you alive. I am continually asked about vitamin and mineral intake on a plant-based diet and whether I get all that I need. A well-planned plant-based diet will give you all you need, even more than anyone eating a typical Western diet, thanks to all of the veggies, fruits, nuts, seeds, legumes and gluten-free whole grains bursting with vitamins, minerals, antioxidants and fibre to balance your system.

Vitamin and mineral supplements are big business, and it seems that far too many people now rely on supplements over a good diet. They can help to correct certain health issues and are vital in some instances, but high-quality real food is what you need to be reaching for before synthetic supplements. Nature has cleverly designed foods to deliver the nutrients that your body needs in the correct proportions. Vitamins and minerals are important, but it can be dangerous to have too much of a good thing. Always consult a qualified health professional before beginning a course of supplements, as certain nutrients can interact with various medications and cause a risk to your health.

PLANT-BASED EATING AND VITAMIN B12

Vitamin B12 is essential for the protection and growth of the nervous system. If you're not getting enough, you may develop a form of anaemia, fatigue, dizziness, headaches, memory loss and moodiness. It's needed for properly digesting, absorbing and metabolising foods, particularly fats and carbohydrates. One of the only vitamins you need to supplement if you are on a plant-based diet is vitamin B12, as it's found almost entirely in animal protein foods. It's actually synthesised in the soil by bacteria, which animals consume by eating grass. But the fruit and veggies we buy in supermarkets are usually so sanitised that no bacteria or B12 remain.

The body can store vitamin B12 for up to five years, so deficiencies don't become apparent immediately. For this reason, it's a good idea to get your blood B12 levels measured about once a year if you've been on a plant-based diet for five years or more. Vitamin B12 can be found in fortified plant milks, nutritional yeast and some sea vegetables, but my advice is to supplement B12 if you're on a plant-based diet. I use a daily spray under my tongue of methylcobalamin, which is the most effective form of B12 as it gets absorbed straight into the bloodstream.

VITAMIN D: THE SUNSHINE VITAMIN

Vitamin D deficiency is a big problem in colder climates. There are a number of different types of vitamin D, but vitamin D3 (cholecalciferol), which is made in the skin when we're in sunlight, is the most active form and the type that we need to supplement. Spending just 15 minutes in adequate sunlight three times a week ensures that you'll get enough vitamin D. But in the more northern European countries there is not enough sunlight between November and March to make vitamin D3 naturally, so supplementing is important for your immunity and even to prevent depression. Some plant foods contain vitamin D, such as oatmeal, dandelion greens, shiitake and chanterelle mushrooms, sweet potatoes and parsley, plus plant milks like coconut and almond are usually fortified with it. I strongly recommend taking a daily vitamin D3 supplement and avoiding too much sun exposure due to the damage and ageing that UV light can do to your skin.

BEAUTY MINERALS: IRON AND ZINC

Every single cell of your body relies on a constant supply of minerals to stay healthy and to function at their top potential. Minerals are absolutely *essential* for your beauty, vitality and a healthy, fit body, as you can't possibly reach your beautiful best if your cells aren't being fed properly. They're needed for healing and growth throughout the body. A deficiency of just one mineral can imbalance your entire system.

Iron is one of the most talked-about minerals, particularly for women on a plant-based diet. For good reason too, as women need sufficient quantities of the trace mineral throughout their menstruating and child-bearing years. Iron's most important job is to produce haemoglobin in the blood and to oxygenate red blood cells. It helps keep your immune system healthy and gives you plenty of energy for everyday life. A deficiency in iron is called anaemia, and it can cause dry hair, hair loss, serious fatigue, a pale complexion, dizziness and even slowed-down mental abilities.

As with protein, many of us may associate iron with red meat, but there are plenty of wonderful plant sources too. Leafy green vegetables, broccoli, parsley, quinoa, chia seeds, almonds, avocados, beetroot, nutritional yeast, sea veggies, kidney beans, lentils, sesame seeds, prunes, dates and raisins all contain iron. I have made sure to include almost all of these foods in my *Eat Yourself Beautiful* recipes so that it couldn't be simpler to get all the iron you need from your diet.

When eating plant sources of iron (non-heme iron), always aim to pair them with either vitamin C-rich foods like lemon juice or a vinegar like raw apple cider vinegar. These both help to change the iron into a more absorbable form, called ferrous iron. That's why I add lemon juice to the green goddess smoothie on page 218 and to many dips and dressings.

Zinc is another trace mineral needed in minute quantities, but it's vital for health. Your quest for beautiful skin will be affected without enough zinc, as it helps to prevent acne, balance sebum production in oil glands and build protein. It helps to form collagen, that all-important protein for keeping your complexion firm, smooth and wrinkle free. Zinc also boosts your ability to absorb vitamin A, which is another crucial vitamin for glowing skin and bright eyes. Have you ever suffered from peeling, brittle nails with white spots? That can indicate a zinc deficiency, as can hair loss, acne, and cuts and grazes that are slow to heal. So it really is a top beauty mineral. Just like iron, zinc is found in a host of nuts and seeds, veggies and herbs. Some of the best sources are pumpkin seeds, kelp, beans and legumes, mushrooms, pecan nuts, sunflower seeds, nutritional yeast and parsley.

ORGANIC EATING

It's important to choose organic produce as much as possible, as the soil it has been grown in remains rich in the important minerals you need. Organic fruit and veggies have been enabled to grow and develop as nature intended rather than being ripened artificially before they're naturally ready.

This means that they're chemical free, far superior in beautifying nutrients and taste better too. High-quality, nutrient-dense foods build a healthier and more beautiful body.

I understand that for many it's just not financially possible or it can be difficult to source local, organic fruit and veggies. But it's definitely worth it when you do have the option. While pesticides are intended to kill insects, many of them are actually absorbed into our air, soil, water or food supply, and many are synthetic chemicals that are not safe for humans.

You can reduce your exposure as much as possible by avoiding the foods that tend to be the most concentrated sources of pesticide residues. These include animal fats, meat, milk, cheese and eggs. Buying organic produce is ideal, but you can also source local, seasonal produce from farmers and farmers' markets.

It's essential to wash non-organic fruit and vegetables really well, and in some cases removing the skin is a good idea even if it means you're losing out on various nutrients and the extra fibre. But please don't be put off eating plenty of fruit and veg even if it's not organic, as the levels of pesticides in them tend to be much lower than those found in animal products. Also, the antioxidants naturally present in fruit and veggies can help your body to neutralise and excrete the pesticides safely.

BEAUTIFUL HERBS AND SPICES

The powerful medicinal properties of a huge array of herbs have been used for centuries by Native American, Roman, Persian, Egyptian and Hebrew cultures. There are so many different delicious herbs to use for raw and cooked dishes that can help to enhance your health and balance your body. Nature's very own pharmacy can help to build your immune system to prevent illness, regenerate your liver, balance your hormones and adrenal glands, and detoxify your body to build better skin and help shed excess pounds. Mother Nature really is extraordinary!

You can incorporate herbs into your diet in simple ways to improve your beauty and health, and they can also be bought as teas, oils, tinctures and capsules. Lavender oil can be dabbed directly onto spots and blemishes to calm and heal them. Tea tree oil is a powerful antiseptic and antibiotic. Echinacea is brilliant for stimulating your immune system and can help to ward off colds, flu and cold sores, while milk thistle supports the liver in detoxing and aloe vera helps to heal and cleanse your digestive system and soothe inflamed or dry skin.

SPICE UP YOUR LIFE

It's really easy to make herbs and spices a part of your everyday life in the form of teas and by using them in cooking.

Herbal teas offer so many benefits, especially when drunk up to three times a day. I love peppermint tea and ginger tea for reducing bloating, stimulating digestion and soothing the digestive tract. Chamomile tea calms your system and is excellent for inducing sleep at night-time. Liquorice tea helps to improve energy, stamina and the function of your thyroid, dandelion tea is effective for its diuretic properties and warming cinnamon tea improves poor circulation. Herbal teas can help you to drop water weight before a big event by stimulating your kidneys to expel more fluid. I often drink dandelion tea for a few days before a big shoot or a red carpet event in order to feel my very best.

THE *EAT YOURSELF BEAUTIFUL* GUIDE TO HERBS AND SPICES

I have tried to incorporate the most healing herbs and spices into as many of my *Eat Yourself Beautiful* recipes as possible. Many of them will be pantry cupboard staples and even firm favourites already, but here's a handy guide to choosing which are right for you.

CARDAMOM
Reduces gas, bloating and irritable bowel syndrome.

CAYENNE PEPPER
Boosts metabolism and circulation and improves blood flow.

CINNAMON
Stimulates circulation, reduces bloating and gas, boosts digestion and its chromium content helps to improve sugar metabolism.

CLOVES
Antiseptic, antimicrobial and reduces nausea, gas and bloating. It can also be applied topically for toothache.

FENNEL
Freshens breath and prevents gas and bloating.

GARLIC
The important chemical in garlic is alliin, which is converted to allicin. It's activated by air and denatured by heat, so chopping raw garlic and leaving it in the air for a few minutes before consuming it is the best way to avail of its healing properties. Garlic helps to lower blood pressure and cholesterol, thins out blood and acts as an anti-inflammatory, antioxidant and antifungal. Don't mind the garlic breath!

GINGER
Anti-inflammatory, boosts circulation and eases nausea, bloating and abdominal discomfort.

MUSTARD
Helps to boost poor circulation and digestion.

OREGANO
Antioxidant, antimicrobial, fights candida and reduces nausea, gas, bloating, digestive imbalance, fungal infections and chest infections.

PARSLEY
Removes gas, bloating and water retention. A powerful antioxidant, it's also rich in vitamins C and K.

PEPPER
Improves poor circulation and weak digestion. Increases the availability of nutrients from foods and other spices, especially turmeric.

PEPPERMINT
Reduces gas and bloating, is antimicrobial, has mildly sedative effects and reduces nausea.

ROSEMARY
Reduces bloating and excess gas, improves poor circulation.

SAGE
Antimicrobial and antibiotic. Improves poor memory and concentration.

THYME
Antioxidant, anti-parasitic, antifungal and antimicrobial. Clears mucus from the lungs and eases chest infections, coughs, diarrhoea and bad breath.

TURMERIC
Reduces inflammation, brightens skin, thins blood and boosts liver and digestive health.

SALT: ONE OF THE ULTIMATE BEAUTY-BUSTERS

Have you ever noticed that some people have very dark circles around their eyes, a puffy face and bags under their eyes that don't go away no matter how much sleep they get? A common cause is a diet too high in sodium chloride (salt) and too low in potassium. Even the best concealer can't hide a less-than-healthy intake of salt. Unfortunately, most packaged sweet and savoury processed foods are full of added salt. An excessive intake of salt and low amounts of potassium in the diet really strain your kidneys' job in preserving a healthy fluid volume in your blood and show up as circles, puffiness and blood stagnating under your eyes. This can create high blood pressure and water retention, making people look pounds heavier than they really ought to. It can also add years to your age and rob you of your healthy glow, as your dehydrated body is struggling to balance itself. The best way to avoid this is by reducing your salt intake and increasing the amount of potassium in your diet. Avoiding most processed foods and eating plenty of fruit and vegetables will naturally resolve the issue. Read food labels carefully to keep your salt intake to 4g or less per day for an adult.

ALCOHOL

To look and feel your most beautiful, healthy and lean, alcohol must be drunk in moderation. I do understand how difficult it can be, as so many of our culture's social occasions, celebrations and feast days involve alcohol and there can be enormous pressure to drink along with everybody else. A glass of red wine does have various health benefits. Most notably, it contains the powerful antioxidant resveratrol, which may protect against heart disease and cancers. But taken in excess, even red wine will contribute to faster ageing. If possible, choose organic wines with no sulphites added. I tend to avoid wine because I'm sensitive to the sulphites, sugar and yeasts in it, but wine is slightly gentler on the liver and other organs than spirits. The most damaging kind of alcoholic drinks you can have are those that have been brewed, such as beer. These are instantly absorbed into the bloodstream, causing a sudden spike in insulin and imbalances in blood sugar levels. Their sugars also encourage the growth of unfriendly bacteria and yeasts in the digestive system, leading to bloating.

It's always a good idea to drink a glass of water for every alcoholic drink you have and to be mindful about the speed you're drinking at. It takes one hour for your body to metabolise a unit of alcohol, so you should choose your own pace and not be pressured into having more than you intended to.

LINING THE STOMACH

Before a night out, make sure you eat a meal or snack with plenty of protein, fibre and healthy fats to line your stomach and give you long-lasting energy. Mashed avocado on seeded gluten-free toast, chopped apple with almond butter or even a good handful of raw almonds can really help. Skipping food to allow for alcohol calories is a really bad idea, because a night of drinking the simple carbs in alcohol will mess with your blood sugar levels so much that you crash the following day and will be more likely to binge on sugary, salty and fatty foods to restabilise your blood electrolytes.

CHOCOLATE IS A BEAUTY FOOD

In its raw, unprocessed state, chocolate is a true beauty food. Eaten in moderation, chocolate desserts and sweet treats can help you to stay on track with a healthy lifestyle. The *Eat Yourself Beautiful* desserts are all free from gluten, dairy, refined sugar and other processed ingredients, and in many cases are raw and filled with living enzymes. There are few greater pleasures than preparing tasty treats for family and friends, and it's even better when they support your beauty and body goals too. My aim is for you to find the desserts and treats in this book so satisfying that you won't even notice that toxic ingredients are missing.

Dark chocolate is my favourite treat because it contains heart-healthy fats and polyphenols called flavonoids. In fact, it's one of the best sources of antioxidants of any food in the world. I have used raw cacao in many of the dessert recipes in this book because it's minimally processed, high in vitamins B and C, fibre and antioxidants to protect your skin from ageing and high in minerals such as iron, zinc, copper, calcium and magnesium. The nutrients in raw chocolate have also been shown to lower blood pressure, boost blood circulation and cardiovascular health, suppress appetite and improve production of digestive enzymes. Raw cacao is also thought to be an aphrodisiac and the ancient Aztecs believed chocolate was the food of the heart, so some of the desserts and sweet treats would be perfect to make for a romantic night in! However, cacao is also a stimulant as it contains theobromine and caffeine, so it's best to enjoy it in smaller amounts and not every day.

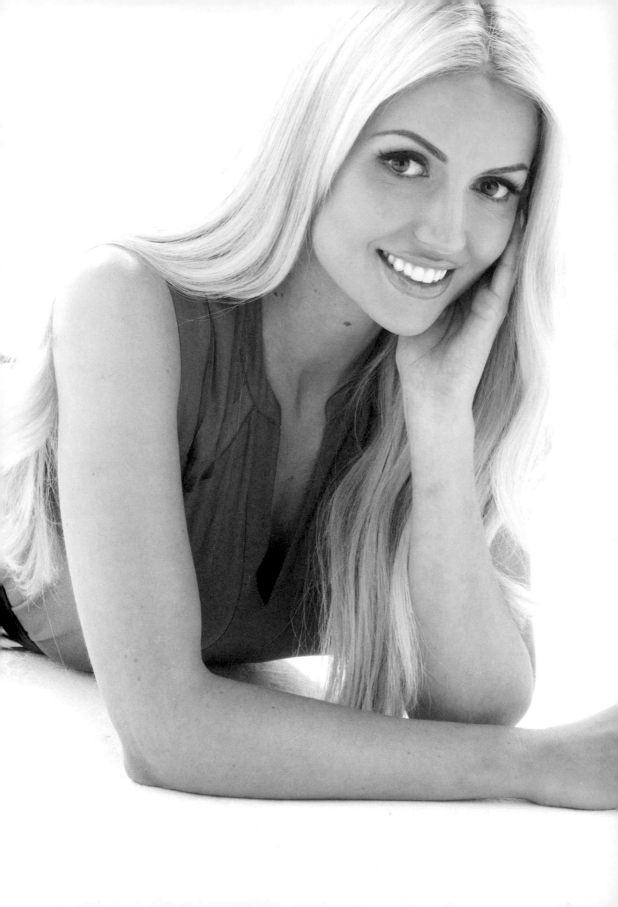

BEAUTIFUL SKIN, HAIR AND BODY

'WE HAVE FAR MORE CONTROL OVER OUR HEALTH AND THE CONDITION OF OUR BODIES THAN WE EVER THOUGHT POSSIBLE.' *Mike Rabe*

BEAUTIFUL SKIN

From the ancient Egyptians to cultures around the world today, smooth, supple, youthful skin is a beauty trend that has never gone out of fashion. We spend more money on make-up, skincare and treatments created to make our skin look better than on any other type of cosmetic. Many of these products do work well to clean off make-up and grime and to protect skin from dryness and environmental damage. For instance, I'm obsessed with wearing a daily SPF 50 moisturiser. But there's only so much a cream or serum can do when your skin cells have already been built.

There is a powerful connection between your food and your beauty. As Dr Georgianna Donadio, founder of the National Institute of Whole Health, explains, 'Your skin is the fingerprint of what is going on inside your body, and all skin conditions, from psoriasis to acne to ageing, are the manifestations of your body's internal needs, including its nutritional needs.'

By making changes to what you eat, you can dramatically alter how you look. What you eat literally becomes you and it is so much more effective to nourish skin from within as your skin cells and the collagen that forms your skin's structure are all being built. Think about what would be most effective: rubbing oil on the outer layers of your skin in the hope that it can prevent wrinkles, or lubricating and nourishing the skin from its very formation with essential fats so that the cell walls are supple and strong and your collagen framework holds everything firmly together. The latter is how you can prevent dryness, sagging and wrinkles from forming. No cream will ever compare to what the right foods will do for building beautiful skin.

The skin is our largest organ for detoxification. It also tells you a lot about the inner workings of your body and the health of your blood, organs and systems. A diet high in processed foods, animal fats, sugar and dehydrating alcohol and caffeine will usually show up as a dull complexion and dark circles under the eyes, no matter how much sleep you get. Dull skin, pimples and premature wrinkles are unfortunately a very common problem. Treating skin issues with *functional nutrition*, using a whole foods, plant-based diet, with extra focus placed on the vitamins, minerals and foods for youthful skin, is the most powerful way to get a glowing complexion.

SAY GOODBYE TO ACNE

Traditionally thought of as a teenage problem, adult acne also affects thousands of people. I suffered from teenage breakouts, particularly hormonal ones, but when I continued to get breakouts of swollen red spots in my twenties, I began to understand the link between diet and skin. The breakouts often happened after work trips and holidays abroad, when my usually balanced diet was compromised by airplane food, tempting buffet desserts, ice creams and the bread basket at restaurants. After eliminating various foods and keeping a strict food diary, I discovered that dairy, wheat and sugar were the culprits behind my breakouts. Since cutting the terrible trio out of my life, healing my digestive system, adding probiotics and alkalising my body with nutritious plant foods, those painful pimples have gone for good too. The *Eat Yourself Beautiful* plan is designed to balance your hormones as much as possible, regulate your cycle and minimise premenstrual symptoms. Changing my diet has literally changed my life, and that's what I'm hoping this way of eating will do for you too.

THE *EAT YOURSELF BEAUTIFUL* GUIDE TO GETTING RID OF ACNE

1

Eating a diet high in raw fruit and vegetables and low in white flour and processed foods dramatically lowers levels of acne. All processed foods must be avoided, including refined salt.

2

A high-fibre diet is crucial for keeping your digestive tract clean and clear of acne-causing toxic waste.

3

Zinc is an important mineral for healing your skin and improving immune system health. Some cases of acne may be a sign of zinc deficiency. Zinc is antibacterial and is needed in your skin's oil glands. Eat plenty of zinc-rich foods, such as pumpkin and sunflower seeds, spinach, beans and mushrooms.

4

Probiotics improve gut health, the function of your liver and immune system and they increase your digestion and ability to absorb nutrients for clear, healthy skin.

5

Vitamins C, E and A are essential for clear, healthy skin. The *Eat Yourself Beautiful* recipes all include foods like berries, peppers, almonds, sesame seeds, avocados, sweet potatoes and butternut squash, which are rich in vitamins C, E and A.

6

Essential fatty acids, like omega-3, are absolutely crucial for clearing up acne and building smooth, supple skin. As most of us tend to be deficient in omega-3 fats rather than omega-6, aim to eat chia seeds, hemp seeds, walnuts and ground flaxseed regularly.

7

Water, water, water! H_2O is the quickest way to flush toxins out of your body, clear up your skin and boost your energy levels. Aim to drink at least eight glasses every day.

8

For clearing up acne, avoid wheat and gluten, dairy, meat, poultry, fried foods, saturated and trans fats, caffeine, fizzy drinks, sugar and junk foods. It's easier than you might think to change food habits, especially when you start to see positive results.

9

It's important to avoid all types of sugar, including fruit juice, when healing acne, as it attacks your white blood cells and debilitates your immune system. It also feeds candida, another cause of acne.

10

Keep skin clean and free from excess oils and wash your hair regularly. Sleep on a clean pillow, use clean face towels and try to use natural skincare and mineral-based make-up. Avoid any temptation to squeeze your spots.

11

Avoid excess stress as much as you can. I know this isn't always easy, but if stress hormones are regularly circulating in your system, it can alter your hormonal balance, which can lead to acne breakouts.

BEAUTIFUL SKIN FOODS

To make life easier in the supermarket, I have divided the best skin foods into four main categories: fruit, vegetables, fats and important others.

BEAUTY FRUIT

While all fruits are rich in collagen-building vitamin C, I have selected each of the following for their unique health and beauty benefits.

APPLES

Their copper helps you to produce melanin, the pigment responsible for colour in your skin. This protects your skin from UV rays and helps to build healthy tissues, hair and eyes.

BERRIES

Rich in antioxidants called anthocyanins and quercetin to keep your skin strong, smooth and youthful.

FIGS

Their high fibre content stimulates digestion, eliminates waste, dissolves mucus and supports the growth of friendly bacteria, including *acidophilus*, which leads to clearer skin.

LEMONS

Improve digestion and give you clear, luminous skin by boosting your liver's bile secretion and supporting your its detox enzymes. Lemons are also rich in the alkalising minerals magnesium, potassium and calcium.

MANGO

Rich in beta-carotene, which repairs and renews your skin cells and mucus membranes and protects your skin from UV damage.

PEARS

An excellent source of the antioxidant vitamins A, C and E for beautiful skin, plus a range of essential skin minerals like selenium, zinc and copper as well as pectin, a soluble fibre.

PINEAPPLE

Contains a special proteolytic enzyme called bromelain, which helps to break down the protein in the food you eat, supports digestion, stimulates your digestive enzymes and clears toxins from your blood.

BEAUTY VEGETABLES

All whole, unprocessed vegetables will do wonders for your skin, hair and body, but I love the following for their benefits, taste and versatility in recipes.

BROCCOLI

High in calcium, copper, zinc, potassium and the ACE group of vitamin antioxidants to fight free radical damage and build collagen. Broccoli contains glucoraphanin, which gets converted into sulforaphane, a phytonutrient shown to protect cells from UV damage.

BUTTERNUT SQUASH

A serious skin-glow food and an excellent source of beta-carotene, which is crucial for your skin's health and integrity. Their vitamin C prevents fine lines, wrinkles, pigmentation and sagging.

CABBAGE

Their rich vitamin A, C and E levels and sulphur help to build younger-looking skin, reduce wrinkles and cleanse toxins from your blood, including free radicals and uric acid, which can create lines and other signs of ageing.

CARROTS

Another great source of beta-carotene to protect and repair skin tissue and to lessen damage from the sun's rays.

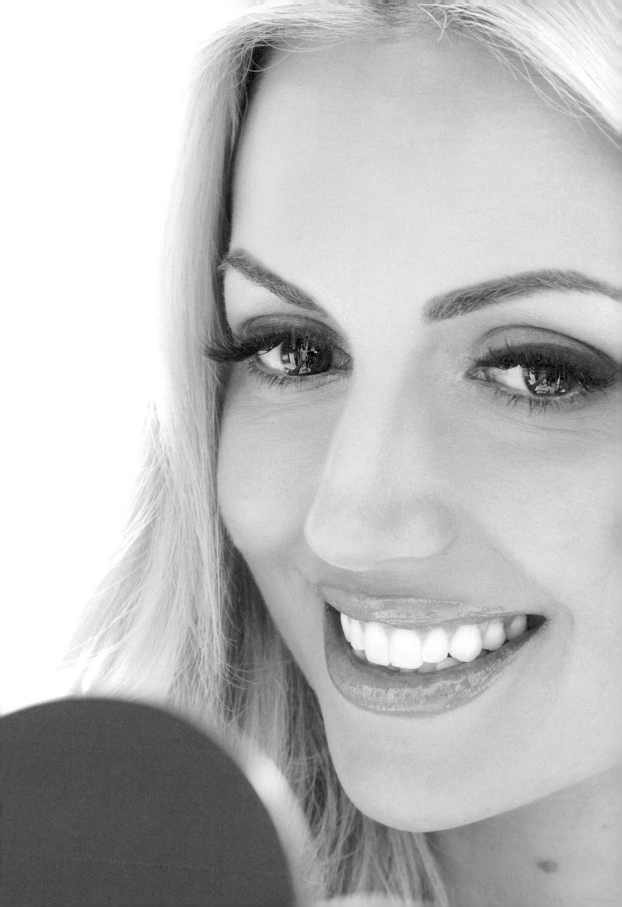

CUCUMBER

A key source of vitamin C, beta-carotene, silica and manganese for beautiful skin, plus alkalising water and electrolytes to hydrate cells and keep skin looking plump and fresh. Their caffeic acid also helps to reduce fluid retention and inflammation.

RED PEPPERS

Packed with more than twice the vitamin C of citrus fruits to increase your skin's ability to fight the damage caused by free radicals, red peppers also contain silicon to increase your skin's suppleness, reduce fine lines and wrinkles and prevent sagging skin. All bell peppers are a great source of vitamins A, C and K, but the red ones also boast carotenoids such as lycopene to prevent premature ageing.

SPINACH

High levels of beta-carotene and lipoic acid aid in rejuvenating the skin-promoting antioxidant vitamins C and E. Spinach also contains zinc and selenium for youthful-looking skin and beauty minerals like iron, calcium, potassium, magnesium, copper, choline, B vitamins for energy and skin-smoothing omega-3 fatty acids.

TOMATOES

Tomatoes have high amounts of antioxidants, including the four main carotenoids (alpha- and beta-carotene, lutein and lycopene), which work together to provide powerful anti-ageing health benefits. Lycopene has the strongest antioxidant capacity of all the carotenoids, helping to scavenge the free radicals that cause lines, wrinkles and other signs of premature ageing and protecting your skin from UV damage.

BEAUTY FATS

Good fats are essential to lubricate, soften and nourish your body and skin from the inside out. Here are my top choices.

ALMONDS

A great source of plant protein and one of the best food sources of vitamin E to nourish, soften and protect your skin from sun damage.

AVOCADO

One of the very best food sources of potassium and the beautifying ACE vitamins, plus iron and copper, the mineral components of antioxidant enzymes. Avocados also include the protective amino acids glutamine and glutathione. Studies have shown that glutathione helps to slow down ageing.

CHIA SEEDS

One of the very highest sources of omega-3 fats to nourish your skin and keep your cell membranes strong and supple. Chia seeds are loaded with antioxidants to protect your skin from free radical damage, are rich in potassium and iron and have five times more calcium than milk.

COCONUT

The electrolytes in coconut water are similar to our blood. They rehydrate you, helping to plump up skin. The powerful antibacterial and antifungal properties in all forms of coconut protect skin from breakouts and infections.

FLAXSEEDS

Flaxseeds have the perfect essential fatty acid balance, plus calcium, magnesium, iron, zinc, folate, manganese and B6. Flaxseeds are also high in soluble and insoluble fibre to keep blood sugar levels stable and sweep toxins and old hormones out of your intestines. This cleanses the body of waste products and allows nutrients to better reach your skin.

HEMP SEEDS

A powerhouse of all the essential amino acids, B vitamins, calcium, iron, dietary fibre, the protective skin vitamins A and E and an ideally balanced ratio of omega-6 to omega-3 fats to boost cell membranes and protect against inflammation.

PUMPKIN SEEDS

Rich in zinc, which keeps collagen strong, helps skin to renew itself and protects your cell membranes from damage.

SUNFLOWER SEEDS

Full of vitamin E to neutralise cell-damaging free radicals and anti-inflammatory to reduce the risk of acne and psoriasis. A rich source of selenium, a powerful antioxidant nutrient that helps vitamin E to repair your DNA. Sunflower seeds are also a good source of fibre, B vitamins for energy, folate, phosphorus, amino acids for growth and repair of your skin and essential fatty acids for smooth skin.

WALNUTS

Their omega-3 fats strengthen your skin cell membranes and lock in moisture and nutrients to keep it looking youthful, plump and glowing. Plus they reduce the inflammation that leads to breakouts, which means fewer spots.

IMPORTANT OTHERS

GARLIC

Antifungal and antibacterial, garlic also contains skin-beautifying minerals like zinc, sulphur, calcium and selenium. Due to its salicylate, garlic thins blood and boosts blood flow, which brings more nutrients to your skin to make it glow.

ONIONS

An excellent anti-inflammatory blood cleanser, onions are packed with quercetin, calcium, potassium, iron, silicon and the ACE group of protective antioxidant vitamins.

RAW APPLE CIDER VINEGAR

Promotes blood circulation in the tiny capillaries that deliver nutrients to your skin. It also prevents growth of the bacteria, yeasts and viruses that can cause infections and is a powerful digestion booster. Its antifungal, antiviral and antibacterial powers rebalance your intestinal flora, which helps to reduce pesky sugar cravings.

TURMERIC

Its antioxidant flavonoid, curcumin, helps to boost blood circulation, deliver more nutrients to skin, cleanse blood and heal damaged cells.

SAY GOODBYE TO BAGS UNDER YOUR EYES

Who doesn't get bags under their eyes when they're seriously tired, jet-lagged, overworked and under-slept? I certainly do! For a lot of people, their dark under-eye bags continue to plague them even if they're getting eight hours of sleep a night. Unfortunately, there is a much deeper reason for dark, puffy eyes than a lack of sleep: diet plays an enormous part in reducing and even eliminating those dark circles and puffy bags. Dehydration, smoking and too many salty foods can all lead to dark circles under your eyes. But the leading reason for them developing is when the adrenal system is under too much pressure. This can be from too much caffeine, refined carbs, alcohol, poor sleep and general stress and anxiety. While you can't always control what stressors come into your life, you can certainly support your delicate adrenal glands in their important function by eating plenty of whole plant foods, managing stress levels, staying hydrated and cutting down on processed, refined or deep-fried foods.

DARK CIRCLES AND YOUR KIDNEYS

It's normal to see dark circles accompanied by puffiness around the delicate area under the eyes. This is generally related to kidney function, and too much sodium (and alcohol) cause big problems. It's really important to cut down on salty foods and to increase your intake of potassium-rich foods for kidney function to return to normal and stored fluids to be flushed out of your cells. Eating water-rich plant foods should help to rebalance your body and banish those bags. I refer to these foods as diuretics, as they're cleansing agents that release stored fluid from your body. They do this by encouraging more sodium to be excreted in your urine, which pulls water from your tissues and cells. Sure, you can buy over-the-counter pharmaceutical diuretics, but save your hard-earned cash and fill up on natural diuretic foods instead while benefitting from all of their anti-ageing nutrients at the same time.

UNDER-EYE BEAUTY FOODS

These are some of the best foods for a smooth and even under-eye area.

ASPARAGUS

Extremely effective in diminishing bloating in your body as well as puffiness under your eyes. Asparagus contains 288 milligrams of potassium per cup and is naturally low in salt, which balances out your blood electrolytes, boosts kidney function and banishes bloat.

BANANAS

Their potassium balances out blood electrolyte levels, encouraging your cells and kidneys to flush out stored water and reduce under-eye puffiness. High in magnesium, bananas help to make you feel more relaxed and calm a taxed adrenal system, which is a major cause of under-eye darkness.

CELERY

With the ideal balance of potassium and natural sodium, stored-up bodily fluids are flushed out via your kidneys to reduce water retention in your abdomen, ankles and under the eyes. Celery contains a bioactive compound, polyacetylene, which is anti-inflammatory to help balance your system.

GINGER

Helps to improve blood flow and can prevent blood from stagnating under your eyes, creating those dark shadows that are difficult to conceal. Ginger is highly anti-inflammatory due to its compounds called gingerols and is great for puffiness under your eyes. It also works well as a diuretic.

BEAUTIFUL HAIR

The cellular and metabolic processes that build healthy, strong and shiny locks depend on a well-balanced and nutrient-rich diet. A sugar, alcohol or fatty food binge can reveal itself pretty quickly in your complexion and in the area under your eyes, causing spots, excess oil, dry patches or water retention, but it can take a little longer for the effects of a nutrient deficiency or a poor diet to really show themselves in your hair. This also applies to positive changes in diet and lifestyle, so you need to be a little more patient with hair growth. However, I really noticed that my hair became softer, shinier, longer and healthier when I started drinking the green goddess smoothie on page 218 every day and added kale salads and homemade kale crisps (page 238) to my diet.

Each strand of your hair grows from the follicle and the surrounding scalp, which are nourished by the foods you eat and the nutrients you absorb into your blood and cells. A healthier scalp and follicles equals healthier, shinier and stronger hair. While a good diet is essential, a lack of sleep, imbalanced hormones and smoking can reverse these good effects. Crash diets and restrictive dieting are bad for your overall health, but they also affect your hair's health. Your body doesn't consider your hair to be essential for survival, so if you have a nutrient deficiency, all the available nutrients are directed towards your vital organs instead.

Since hair is nearly 100% protein, getting the right amino acids from the foods you eat is vital for a beautiful head of hair. Just as intestinal congestion, constipation or a toxic build-up will affect your skin's health, a digestive tract working less than optimally will affect the type and quantity of hair-boosting nutrients you absorb. Foods that can block up your body and create irritation, mucus, toxins and unfriendly bacteria growth include animal fats, dairy, soy products, wheat and gluten, sugar, alcohol and cooked vegetable oils. The type of continuous detox eating plan in *Eat Yourself Beautiful* supports intestinal, blood, tissue, cell and lymphatic cleansing and enables nutrients to reach your hair follicles via the tiny blood capillaries in your scalp.

BEAUTIFUL HAIR FOODS

Here are some of the best foods for healthy hair. I love the fact that most are inexpensive and easy to find in good supermarkets.

LENTILS

Jam-packed with healthy hair nutrients like fibre, iron, biotin, zinc and complete protein, one cup of cooked lentils provides almost 18g of protein and only 0.8g of fat.

NUTRITIONAL YEAST

A form of inactive yeast grown on molasses and cane sugar, nutritional yeast is suitable for anyone who is sensitive to yeast or suffering from *Candida albicans* overgrowth. It contains the ideal mix of your hair's most important nutrients, and is rich in 18 different amino acids to strengthen hair growth and B vitamins, including biotin.

PUMPKIN SEEDS

One of the best foods for building strong, shiny hair and a good source of zinc, sulphur and vitamin A for follicular health. Their vitamins C and E keep your scalp moisturised with sebum and protect your cells from oxidative damage. The biotin and 15.6g of protein per serving in pumpkin seeds boosts the growth of strong, healthy hair.

QUINOA

Full of essential amino acids, which are needed for hair growth, healthy skin and sexy, toned muscles, quinoa is also one of the best plant sources of the amino acid lysine, which is crucial for tissue growth, the synthesis of collagen and elastin and the repair of damaged cells. The calcium, iron and phosphorus in quinoa help to prevent dandruff and seal moisture into your scalp, while its vitamin E keeps each strand soft and supple. It contains tyrosine, which is the parent amino acid for your hair, skin and eye pigment, and helps to maintain your original hair colour.

SPINACH

Packed with easily absorbed and assimilated amino acids, iron, vitamins A, C and E, folate, beta-carotene and other phytonutrients and antioxidant minerals like zinc and selenium to renew call growth and keep your scalp and follicles fed with a nourishing blood supply.

SWEET POTATO

A great source of beta-carotene, sweet potato supports and nourishes the cells in your scalp by helping to produce the conditioning and moisturising oils that build vibrant hair.

WALNUTS AND BRAZIL NUTS

An excellent source of zinc, a handful of walnuts a day will really boost hair condition. Brazil nuts are full of biotin and the antioxidant mineral selenium, which are important for hair growth and your scalp's health.

ACHIEVING YOUR IDEAL BODY WEIGHT

We're all familiar with the word *obesity*. It's defined as an excessive amount of body fat, with a body mass index (BMI) over 30 and a body fat percentage greater than 30% for women and 25% for men. The obesity epidemic of the modern Western world is a perfectly predictable physiological response by the human body to our sedentary lifestyles and the foods we consume.

But obesity is a far more complex issue than just what you eat and how often you exercise. There is a variety of hormones working closely together that regulate weight, fat storage, hunger and satisfaction after eating in people within the healthy weight range. It's in your body's best interests to maintain a balanced metabolism and level of fat storage so that equilibrium can be achieved at all times. It also means that you're driven to eat a similar quantity of calorific energy each day, stopping when you're no longer hungry, so your weight shouldn't fluctuate excessively.

So why does this delicately balanced system fail an increasing number of people? Weight gain can be an incredibly complex situation, involving both physiological and psychological factors, like emotional eating and food cravings. In many cases, the physiological reasons behind excess fat storage are insulin resistance due to a diet high in sugar and processed carbs, changes to your appetite-signalling hormones, a change in how food is burned for energy and low levels of brain serotonin, which leads to more sugar cravings. It's a vicious cycle that can be extremely challenging to break.

FAT AROUND THE MIDDLE

The love handles and inner thigh fat stores that many of us struggle with may be frustratingly tough to get rid of, but if you're within the normal weight range, they're not a health risk. However, abdominal fat is the type stored around the midriff, which can create a cascade of problems for the entire metabolism and hormonal system. Measuring my client's waist-to-hip ratio (ideally 1 for men and less than 0.8 for women), waist size and waist-to-height ratio are a mandatory part of my consultation because waist size and how it compares to hips and height can tell us a lot about current and future health risks. Ideally, your waist should be less than 37 inches for men and 31.5 inches for women and your waist must always remain less than half your height.

INSULIN

Insulin is produced by the pancreas and released into the bloodstream, where it's responsible for controlling blood sugar (glucose) levels. It's our fat storage hormone and it is critical to the body's ability to use glucose for energy. High levels of glucose in the bloodstream signal an abundance of energy. This is swiftly shunted into our cells by insulin, where it's either used as immediate energy or stored as fat in the stomach area so the liver can access it quickly for instant energy.

CORTISOL

Cortisol is one of the stress hormones, produced in the adrenal glands that sit above the kidneys. It works closely with insulin in storing fat around the middle. The fat around our middle also works as an endocrine gland, producing a large amount of hormones and other substances that actually alter metabolism, cause us to lose track of our hunger signals and reach for sugary and fatty foods. Therefore, fat around the abdomen doesn't just sit quietly like fat in other parts of the body. It produces its own chemicals that cause us to want to eat more. A stressful lifestyle coupled with a high-sugar and processed carb diet is the perfect recipe for fat storage around the middle. When both insulin and cortisol are raised for an extended period of time, you develop fat around the middle, an increase in appetite and an urge for chocolate, bread, biscuits, caffeine and alcohol. They cause that familiar mid-afternoon slump and further cravings. Together they also lower your immune system and cause fatigue, mood swings, muscle and joint aches, digestive difficulties and poor memory and concentration. Do any of these problems sound familiar? Working in tandem, insulin and cortisol can destroy your health, make you age faster and make it much more difficult to manage your weight.

TOO MUCH FOOD, TOO FEW NUTRIENTS

Obese children and adults are some of the most malnourished people in modern society. One of the biggest dietary misconceptions out there is that the more food and calories we consume, the more nourished we will be, but this couldn't be further from the truth.

How can these opposite states co-exist? Eating the standard Western diet that's high in refined and processed foods actually increases our biological need for vitamins and minerals. These nutrients are required to feed the various metabolic cycles that keep us alive. The big issue is that this typical diet is far too rich in empty calories from refined sugar and unhealthy fat and too low in the essential nutrients. The nutrients we do get are used to process and metabolise toxic foods, leaving little left over to tend to normal bodily needs. Most modern processed food is horribly low in nutrients. Humans evolved on fresh, local, seasonal, nutrient-rich foods that didn't require processing, chemicals, artificial colours and preservatives. If you're eating plenty but your body isn't getting the vitamins and minerals it needs to survive, it will keep calling out for food, which you start to interpret as needing high-energy foods like stodgy carbs and chocolate.

DO CALORIES REALLY COUNT?

We live in a society that's growing fatter and sicker by the decade, but remains obsessed with counting calories. If maintaining your weight was as simple as the diet industry and mainstream media make it out to be, then we'd all be slender and glowing with good health. The problem with focusing on calorie consumption is the belief that all calories are created equal. Imagine skipping your dinner of a huge 200 calorie bowl of nourishing veggies for a 200 calorie bowl of ice cream. They each add 200 calories to your body, but they're going to have dramatically different effects once they're broken down and metabolised. The vegetables are so full of fibre that their energy is gradually absorbed, creating no blood sugar spike or insulin rush. But the ice cream will digest quickly, releasing a rush of glucose into your blood. This will trigger a massive insulin response, which is counterproductive for burning fat. The subsequent sugar crash will soon leave you hungry again and craving another sweet hit to boost flagging energy levels. The processed sugar and other artificial ingredients also damage collagen in your skin and lead to premature ageing.

Some types of calories are fattening, some are health promoting and some boost metabolism, while others encourage weight gain. Every single morsel of food you swallow distributes its unique set of information to your system. This information can either support your beauty, weight loss and health goals or it can create accelerated ageing, weight gain and disease.

CALORIES STILL MATTER

But that doesn't mean you can ignore calories completely. There are a number of reasons why keeping an eye on calorie intake is helpful, but it's the tunnel-vision focus on calories as king that I'm very much against. Yes, the type of calories from food matters, but if you regularly eat or drink more calories than you use up, you'll gain weight.

NUTRIENT DENSITY VS. CALORIE DENSITY

The trick to weight loss without counting calories is choosing nutrient density over calorie density. Getting all the nutrients that you need for health and vitality each day while minimising excess energy in the form of empty calories is the ultimate secret to long-term success. It's so simple and effective!

All of my *Eat Yourself Beautiful* recipes are based on nutrient-dense foods. They help to slow down the ageing process, brighten and clear up your complexion, support liver detoxification, increase fat burning and boost bowel health. Their high levels of fibre signal your stomach stretch receptors when you're full. Calorie-dense foods tend to be much lower in healthy nutrients and rich in refined sugar, saturated and trans fats, cholesterol, salt, chemicals and preservatives, which do the opposite of what nutrient-dense foods do for your beauty and body. Whole plant foods are nutrient dense but not calorie dense, and these are the foods that you must aim to really fill up on when you're trying to lose weight.

Foods like nuts, seeds, nut butters and avocados are both nutrient and calorie dense, so to avoid taking in too much energy, it's really important to pay attention to the amount of fat you eat. Plant-based fats are amongst the world's most perfect foods – when eaten in moderation.

Fresh fruit is an excellent nutrient-rich food to eat daily, but be careful with fruit juice and dried fruit if weight loss is your goal, as they have more sugar than fresh fruit.

Alcohol is a classic example of a calorie-dense drink that almost completely lacks nutrients. All alcohol contains 7 calories per gram, which can quickly add up on a night out.

By following the basic principles of filling up on nutrient-dense foods and eating the calorie- and nutrient-dense healthy fats in moderation, I've never found myself thinking about calories or worrying about going over my daily energy intake, especially as I stop eating before I feel stuffed and try not to eat too close to bedtime.

Restrictive diets don't work because they're not a realistic lifestyle and any sort of food restriction will eventually lead to bingeing. That's not because you're greedy or weak. It's simply because as humans built for survival by any means, we're biologically programmed to seek out nourishment and energy in the form of calories.

FOOD CRAVINGS AND LOW SEROTONIN

Serotonin is one of the most important brain neurotransmitters for a positive mental attitude and better-quality sleep. About 80% of the chemical is actually produced in the digestive tract, but low levels in the brain lead to powerful cravings for sugary and stodgy comfort foods.

Tryptophan is the essential amino acid that produces serotonin with the help of co-factors vitamin B6 and zinc. When serotonin drops low, your brain interprets it as a starvation state, which makes you want to quickly fill up on carbs. A high-carbohydrate meal raises insulin levels quickly, which helps to quickly deliver tryptophan past the blood–brain barrier and to the brain, enabling serotonin to be formed. This is what happens to crash dieters who have cut their calorie intake too much and aren't getting their essential nutrients. Their brain sends out an urgent signal to eat a high-carbohydrate meal or snack, which often results in a binge.

On days when a craving for sweet foods hits me, I munch on a handful of organic raisins, raw almonds and pumpkin seeds, and a banana. This works really well, as the raisins create enough of a blood sugar rise to release insulin, but the fat and protein in the nuts slow down the process. Almonds are rich in tryptophan, pumpkin seeds are a good source of zinc and the banana is full of vitamin B6. It's my number one cure for a sugar craving. Regular exercise, avoiding stimulants and excessive alcohol and getting sufficient sleep keep serotonin levels stable and reduce the chances of food cravings.

THE CELLULITE FIGHT

Oh, cellulite. Unique to us ladies, it's estimated that 80–90% of women have cellulite. It seems to be one of our most disliked physical realities and millions have been made by cosmetics companies convincing us to buy their anti-cellulite creams.

The first time I spied cellulite on the back of my thighs, I was 15 years old and it was the end of a long summer of ice creams and barbecues. Once I got back to my regular exercise routine, a healthy diet and lost the extra few pounds, my cellulite disappeared too.

Cellulite is the pitting and bulging of the tissue just below our skin, particularly on our thighs and bottom. Cellulite is really just fat that has pushed up through the spaces between our collagen, making bumps and dimples easily visible. Genetics and ageing can affect how strong or weak your collagen is, but eating the right kinds of food to support and restore collagen as well as resistance training and lowering overall body fat can all make a huge difference to cellulite. Crash diets can actually make cellulite look even worse. Eating a more alkalising diet and adopting a lifestyle that supports your detoxification organs generally allows your body to begin releasing these stored-up toxins into your bloodstream to be eliminated via the kidneys and bladder.

ANTI-CELLULITE FOODS

To get rid of cellulite, follow a diet rich in whole plant foods and low in inflammatory and acid-forming dairy, meat, sugar, caffeine, cooking oils, fizzy drinks, alcohol, chemical sweeteners and preservatives. The foods that help to build and repair the collagen in your skin (bright, colourful berries, juicy fruits and citrus fruits as well as dark green veggies and sweet potatoes) are also the best for strengthening the connective tissue in your thighs to fight cellulite. The antioxidant minerals zinc and selenium, found in nuts, seeds and legumes, can help to fight cellulite by controlling the metabolism of fat in your body. Two of the very best cellulite-fighting foods are coriander and parsley, as they help to remove heavy metals from your body that may get embedded in your fat cells.

TOP 20 TIPS FOR SUCCESSFUL AND SUSTAINED WEIGHT LOSS

It's really important to remember that you can only lose one or two pounds of *body fat* per week. Any more than that is stored glycogen, muscle mass and water. Losing a little water weight is perfectly okay and will naturally happen when you begin eating a diet rich in nutrients and fibre. But it's crucial that you don't lose your muscle mass by crash dieting or depriving your body of adequate amino acids, because your body will start to break down muscle fibres to be used for energy. Muscle at rest burns far more calories than fat at rest, so maintaining and even building your muscle while focusing on losing extra fat is the best way to ensure a healthy and manageable weight for life.

1
FORGET DIETING

The diet industry has surged by 200% in the past eight years, and its success is based on the fact that diets are designed to fail us. It's inevitable that weight will return when you begin to eat normally again after a restrictive or crash diet, as they're simply not sustainable. When restricting food, your metabolism may slow right down because it sees the decrease in energy as a famine state and will try to preserve calories. This will hamper weight loss efforts and cause fat to pile on when the diet comes to an end. The only way to achieve real and sustained weight loss and glowing health for life is to overhaul an unhealthy diet and lifestyle with nutrient-dense foods and regular exercise.

2
EAT LITTLE AND OFTEN

Eating six smaller meals or snacks every three to four hours throughout the day can really help to keep your blood sugar stable, which in turn means you won't reach for high-fat or high-sugar snacks.

3
NEVER SKIP BREAKFAST

If you're in a rush in the mornings, make a green goddess smoothie (page 218) the night before and pour it into individual bottles to take with you in the morning. You could also make a quick jar of chia pudding or overnight oats to grab from the fridge.

4

ELIMINATE SUGAR AND REFINED CARBOHYDRATES

Simple carbs like sugar, fruit juice, soft drinks, alcohol and white flour raise blood insulin levels, leading to impaired fat burning, weight gain and even insulin resistance over time. Stick to pieces of whole fruit, vegetables, starchy veggies, gluten-free oats and grains instead.

5

EAT PROTEIN WITH EACH MEAL

Add high-fibre protein to each meal or snack, such as a spoonful of nut butter, a handful of almonds or hemp seeds, a serving of nutritional yeast or a few tablespoons of quinoa, sprouted beans or lentils to maintain steady energy levels for the whole day and to ensure you get all your essential amino acids.

6

EAT FATS IN MODERATION

Healthy fats are essential, but it's important not to go overboard with them. Protein and carbohydrates each have 4 calories per gram, but there are 9 calories in every gram of fat, so it can be easy to eat a lot of energy without realising it. Avoid adding oils to food, use low-fat cooking methods like steaming and baking, and be mindful of the quantities of the whole-food fats that you've eaten, like avocado, nuts and olives.

7

SLOW DOWN WHEN YOU EAT AND CHEW YOUR FOOD PROPERLY

Taking the time to chew your food properly and allowing it to mix well with saliva will help it to digest much better in your stomach. Eating slowly also gives your body and brain a chance to register when you're full, which helps to avoid overeating.

8

LIQUIDS COUNT TOO

Fruit juice, soft drinks and creamy cappuccinos all add up throughout the day and can upset appetite-hormone levels. Stick to plain water, herbal teas, green vegetable juice and smoothies or try adding fruit and mint to a jug of chilled water.

9

STOP EATING WHEN YOU'RE THREE-QUARTERS FULL

This is my favourite tip for portion control on a plant-based diet, and it means that counting calories isn't necessary. Low-fat plant-based meals are nutrient dense but low in calorific energy, so you would have to feel seriously stuffed before you overdo it on excess energy. Listening to your body and appetite signals, eating from a smaller plate and finishing when you're three-quarters full will ensure that your weight will stabilise to what is ideal for your body type and height.

10

DON'T EAT WHEN YOU'RE NOT HUNGRY

It's easy to get into the habit of eating out of boredom, or emotional eating. Slowing down, being present in the moment and developing your awareness around food, snacking and the relationship between food and your body make all the difference in achieving your ideal weight.

11

FOCUS ON NUTRIENT-DENSE FOODS

Get used to choosing nutrient-dense plant foods over calorie-dense processed and animal-based foods.

12

STAY HYDRATED

Don't confuse thirst with hunger! Keep a big bottle of water beside you at all times to sip on throughout the day. The only time I'd suggest avoiding water is during a meal, as the extra liquid can dilute your own digestive juices and disrupt the process of digestion. Aim to drink water half an hour before or after meals and plenty during and after exercise.

13

GET ENOUGH SLEEP

Sleep deprivation can trigger low serotonin levels, carbohydrate cravings and weight gain. Aim for at least seven to eight hours of sleep per night to allow your body to grow, heal and renew itself.

14

DON'T EAT OUT TOO OFTEN

It can be difficult to control what you eat in a restaurant, as excess oil, butter, salt and sugar can sneak their way into the food. Ask the waiter for dressings and sauces on the side, for vegetables to be served without butter and for foods to be steamed, not fried.

15

SUPPORT YOUR LIVER

Your liver is your main fat-burning organ, but it can become overwhelmed by excessive alcohol, environmental and dietary chemicals, toxins and cigarette smoke. Support a sluggish liver with detoxifying herbs like milk thistle, cleansing fruit and veggies and plenty of sulphur-rich onions, garlic and cruciferous vegetables.

16

EXERCISE

Try to work up a sweat every day to boost your lymphatic circulation, oxygenate your body and brain, burn stored fat and get those feel-good endorphins pumping. Resistance exercise like weight training really fires up your metabolism long after you have stopped training.

17

BALANCE YOUR HORMONES

Balanced hormones are a key secret to sustained weight loss for life. Excess midriff fat manufactures its own oestrogen, so tackling fat around the middle with the *Eat Yourself Beautiful* programme and regular exercise is essential.

18

WILLPOWER

Nothing will happen without motivation and a positive attitude. For some people a food diary, a photo of themselves, a vision board, a training buddy or an encouraging quote work well. Find your motivational focus and spend a minute or two visualising your goal each morning.

19

BE PRESENT WHILE EATING

Take the time to sit down at the table with your loved ones, enjoy good conversation and appreciate the food in front of you.

20

CHEAT WITH A TREAT

A well-deserved treat helps you to stick to your healthy lifestyle and makes it so much more worth it. Plus it would be bonkers to go through life without tasty treats every so often!

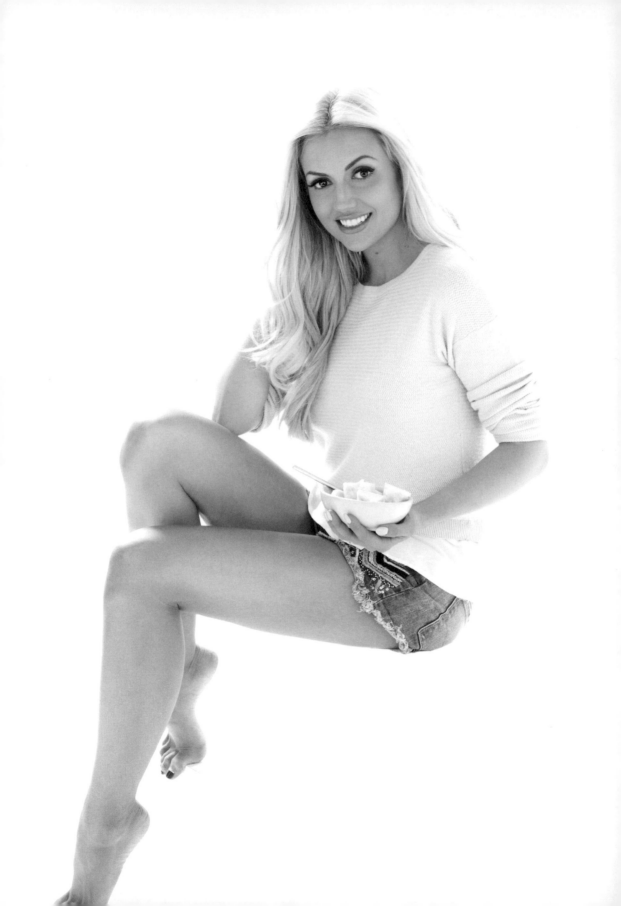

THE *EAT YOURSELF BEAUTIFUL* PROGRAMME

'IT IS HEALTH THAT IS REAL WEALTH AND NOT PIECES OF GOLD AND SILVER.'

Mahatma Gandhi

This chapter is all about how to put the information in the previous chapters into practice. It is the key to combining the foods you eat with your body's natural healing abilities to overhaul your beauty. You need to make your knowledge work for you in your busy life and to see a discernible difference in your body and overall health.

By following the *Eat Yourself Beautiful* programme, you will begin to notice that your skin is glowing, fine lines and wrinkles may start to fade, your hair will grow thicker and shinier, pounds will fall off, your tummy will flatten and dark under-eye circles will diminish. You'll also find that you're sleeping better and enjoying more energy without mid-afternoon slumps and cravings. Moving your vital energy away from the task of digesting oily and meaty meals, wheat and dairy makes all the difference to how you look and feel.

It's so important to listen to your own body and get used to receiving the signals it sends you, such as thirst, hunger, satiety and much more. Being in tune with yourself is one of the great secrets to a lifetime of health. Going from eating a typical diet high in animal protein, refined carbs and cooked oils to an alkalising plant-based diet will cause intense detoxification in your system. Some of these symptoms include aching joints, dizziness, lethargy, skin breakouts, low energy, poor concentration and roller coaster emotions. This is your body dealing with years of stored toxins released from fat cell storage into your bloodstream, and it can often cause people to revert straight back to caffeine and sugar just to feel 'normal' again. They feel 'worse' initially because there are toxins freely circulating in their system when previously they had been safely stored away from vital organs. They may conclude that this type of eating plan isn't for them and that they're deficient in protein or other vitamins and minerals. But it's very difficult to become protein deficient, as amino acids are found in every whole food.

IT'S ALL ABOUT PROGRESS

Making steady progress in the right direction – isn't that what life is about? You have the choice to live a positive life with an optimistic attitude and to build your health in a progressive direction. Some people can overhaul their diet literally overnight, while others prefer to take it in baby steps. Do what works best for you. What counts is moving in the right direction and building your health more each day. Even just adding more plant foods and green smoothies and fewer animal foods to your diet, taking a daily probiotic capsule and substituting plant milk for dairy as often as possible can make a huge difference to how you look and feel. Seeing positive results and feeling lighter, more energetic and less bloated or watching your skin clearing up and beginning to glow will give you that added boost in the right direction. The human body is quick to respond to kinder treatment and it heals

surprisingly fast. When I made the transition from meat-eater to vegetarian to plant-based, it was literally an overnight lifestyle change each time, but I'm an all-or-nothing type. If phasing out less healthy foods is what suits you and your lifestyle, then it's better to move slowly than not at all. However, positive changes to your beauty, body and health will happen more quickly if you do follow my advice as closely as possible.

WHAT IF I MESS UP?

If there's one thing I can guarantee, it's that we will all 'mess up' at some stage. We're only human, and it's inevitable that we will be tempted by less-than-healthy choices throughout our ongoing journey to optimal health. Being mindful of positive self-talk and how you mentally approach temptations really helps. I don't even like to use the term 'mess up' because it places an unnecessarily negative spin on something that is innately human. I try to gently ask myself if I *really* want that 'cheat' food or if I will benefit from it. The answer is generally no. You need to focus on understanding what triggers cravings and how to take back your control over them, following my advice to stabilise blood sugar levels throughout the day and always having a back-up plan for when cravings strike.

So what if you do have a bad day? Health is not built nor destroyed in 24 hours, so you must pick yourself up again, take a deep breath and start fresh. If achieving your health potential was easy, then everybody would do it. You're always going to be challenged by weddings, parties, feast days, holidays and other special occasions, so it's about preparing yourself mentally and physically for a possible onslaught of calorific, blood sugar-spiking and bloating foods and drinks. If you're absolutely starving when you sit down for a meal, it's difficult to refuse a fresh, warm bread roll with lashings of butter. I always eat a snack before a party to make sure I stay well away from the tempting canapés. I have something light but filling with a good mix of digestible protein and healthy fat, like a handful of seeds and berries, a few slices of avocado on wheat-free toast or an apple with a spoonful of nut butter.

If you choose to enjoy a big, greasy treat meal, then you'll likely go to bed feeling bloated, but the next morning you'll be even more inclined to get back on track with a green goddess smoothie (page 218) and some exercise to get your system moving again. This isn't an excuse for it to happen regularly, as unhealthy foods will show up quickly in your skin and on your waistline. But if you do slip up a bit, you'll likely have a strengthened resolve the next day.

THE *EAT YOURSELF BEAUTIFUL* SAMPLE DIET

The one-week sample plan on pages 66–69 represents the ultimate in alkalising, nutrient-dense eating. It will transform your looks and body, and it's the diet that I follow closely myself. You will see the best results if you keep your meals and snacks simple. They needn't take long to prepare, because the most beautifying foods are those that come straight from nature and are virtually unchanged by the time you eat them. As you will see, the plan contains a lot of raw foods, with some comforting cooked dishes to balance it out.

If you're coming from a typical Western diet high in animal foods, dairy, wheat and processed foods, then I recommend that you start off by easing yourself into the *Eat Yourself Beautiful* programme. Remember, this is a way of life, not a quick-fix diet, so

it's perfectly okay to take your time if that's what you need. Start by having a glass of warm water with lemon and a green goddess smoothie in the morning, incorporate more plant foods and fewer animal foods throughout the day, and finish with your normal dinner. Or you may want to have two to three plant-based days a week and eat your normal diet on the other days. Alternatively, you could start by adding the green goddess smoothie and having more dairy-free alternatives. That alone will make a difference to your skin and reduce weight and bloating.

The important thing is to keep adding the healthy foods and reducing the unhealthy foods and drinks in your diet. You will naturally find that within a relatively short space of time, your body will crave more of the clean, fresh foods, and processed sugar, salt and other chemicals will start to taste very unnatural. You should always be actively working to reduce or remove dairy, wheat products, sugar, table salt, fried foods, chemical sweeteners, additives and preservatives, processed and junk foods and cooked vegetable oils from your diet. If you're already used to eating an alkaline diet high in plant foods and just need an extra boost, then you should be well able to follow this programme.

MAKE PLANTS THE MAIN FOCUS

You will see that this plan is bursting with primarily chlorophyll-rich greens and vibrant, colourful vegetables as well as fresh fruit, gluten-free grains, beans and healthy fats. I have included plenty of desserts, sweet treats and indulgent smoothies in the recipe section of the book for special occasions or for times when you want to impress friends and family, and of course to showcase the huge range of delicious guilt-free foods that can be eaten on a plant-based diet. However, if you have been diagnosed with candida or a yeast imbalance, then you need to avoid sweet fruits, dried fruits and sweeteners like honey, molasses and maple syrup.

For the very best beauty results, you must focus mainly on fresh, raw, natural foods. It's important to move away from the mindset that salad and vegetables are just side dishes or garnish. They need to become the *central focus* of your meals, and then you can add other foods to them. I have included plenty of dressings, salsas, hummus and guacamole recipes that you can pile onto salads and steamed or baked veggies to make them interesting and versatile. I hope you'll love the world of flavours that can be created with a few fresh ingredients and store-cupboard staples.

THE *EAT YOURSELF BEAUTIFUL* GUIDE TO PORTION SIZES

Even with some healthy foods, you need to watch how much you're eating to avoid taking in more energy than your body can use. Nutrient-dense rather than calorie-dense foods should be forming the bulk of your diet.

RAW LEAFY GREENS AND COLOURFUL, NON-STARCHY VEGETABLES

These are the most high-nutrient and low-calorie of all the food groups and can be eaten in abundance.

COOKED, NON-STARCHY VEGETABLES

These can also be enjoyed in unlimited amounts when prepared without oil or salt.

FRESH FRUIT

Aim to enjoy ripe, seasonal fruit, washed well before eating. When your body becomes more balanced, up to four servings of fruit a day is perfect. One serving is a medium-sized piece of fresh fruit, and the green goddess smoothie on page 218 contains two to three servings.

STARCH-BASED VEGETABLES

If you're trying to lose weight, then aim to eat just one cup of sweet potato, pumpkin, squash or other starchy vegetable per day. But if you're active or want to maintain your current weight, you can eat more.

RAW NUTS AND SEEDS

If you're trying to lose weight, eat a small handful of nuts or seeds a day. For active people and those maintaining their weight or trying to gain some weight, then two to three handfuls per day is okay.

AVOCADOS

If you're trying to lose weight, eat no more than half a small or medium-sized avocado per day. For everyone else, one full avocado per day is fine.

OIL

All oils should be avoided if you're trying to lose weight, and everybody else should consume oils in strict moderation. Up to 1 tablespoon of coconut oil per day for cooking and baking is acceptable.

GLUTEN-FREE GRAINS

Quinoa, oats, brown rice, millet, buckwheat and amaranth provide you with nutrients and energy. If you're aiming to lose weight, stick to one cup of any of those cooked grains per day. For everyone else, have up to two cups or the amount you feel suits your appetite, activity levels and metabolism.

BEANS AND LEGUMES

These are a high-fibre, low-fat and satisfying food type to help you feel full and keep you well away from fattening snacks. One and a half cups of cooked lentils provide almost 27g of protein and 23.5g of fibre, so one and a half to two cups of cooked lentils, chickpeas or other types of beans and legumes is perfect for active adults. For those trying to lose weight, stick to one cup per day.

ANIMAL PROTEIN (MEAT, POULTRY, FISH, EGGS)

If you decide that you still want to eat animal foods, aim to eat them with your evening meal and up to two to three times a week at most. It's always best to purchase organic, free-range, grass-fed products and wild fish whenever possible. A serving size is equivalent to the size of a deck of cards.

SAMPLE DIET FOR ONE WEEK

You will see that I have included the digestion-boosting basic garden salad (page 108), spicy pineapple salsa (page 146) or raw veggies to be eaten before some of the meals, especially those that involve cooked food, to remind you to boost your digestive enzymes and overall hydration with alkalising greens. It's also a good idea to eat one or two raw Brazil nuts in the morning for their antioxidant nutrient, selenium. Over time, the green goddess smoothie might be enough to satisfy you at breakfast.

The main thing is to listen to your own hunger signals based on your activity levels and metabolic rate, and trust in the power of a whole foods, plant-based diet to transform your beauty and health. Aim to eat until you're three-quarters full and just keep an eye on portions of nuts, nut butters, seeds and avocados, referring to the *Eat Yourself Beautiful* portion guide in the previous section.

All of my breakfast, lunch, dinner, smoothie and savoury snack options are suitable to choose from for three meals and two snacks each day. Try to limit the sweet treats and desserts to a treat at the weekend, as they're higher in energy and can impede weight loss (if that's your goal) if eaten daily. They may be guilt free in that they contain only wholesome ingredients, but they're better viewed as a tasty treat. If you would like to improve your sleep, I have included an optional evening snack rich in tryptophan to be eaten one or two hours before bed.

Finally, sprinkle 2 tablespoons of ground raw flaxseed onto your meals each day to get plenty of essential omega-3 fats.

DAY 1

BREAKFAST

Glass of warm water with the juice of half a lemon followed by a tall glass of green goddess smoothie (page 218)

Creamy berry and coconut quinoa porridge (page 82)

1–2 Brazil nuts

LUNCH

Digestion-boosting basic garden salad (page 108)

Coconut and quinoa curried lentil soup (page 129)

Slice of omega-3 super bread (page 95)

DINNER

Marinated kale, avocado and citrus salad with Rosie's classic salad dressing (page 109)

Blood-cleansing beetroot fries with lemon and parsley hummus (page 145)

SNACKS

Piece of fresh fruit

Handful of raw unsalted nuts and seeds

OPTIONAL EVENING TRYPTOPHAN-RICH SNACK TO BOOST SLEEP

Bedtime banana bites (page 242)

SUPPLEMENTS

Vitamin B12

Probiotic capsule taken after dinner

DAY 2

BREAKFAST

Glass of warm water with the juice of half a lemon followed by a tall glass of green goddess smoothie (page 218)

Cosy apple crumble baked oatmeal (page 94)

1–2 Brazil nuts

LUNCH

Anti-ageing Mauritian salad (page 113)

DINNER

Raw carrots with guacamole (page 152 or page 153)

Roast butternut squash and chickpea stew (page 159)

SNACKS

Pink warrior protein smoothie (page 223)

Fresh fruit

Handful of walnuts or almonds

OPTIONAL EVENING TRYPTOPHAN-RICH SNACK TO BOOST SLEEP

A mug of warm unsweetened almond milk with a pinch of ground cinnamon and a few drops of liquid stevia to sweeten (optional)

SUPPLEMENTS

Vitamin B12

Probiotic capsule taken after dinner

DAY 3

BREAKFAST

Glass of warm water with the juice of half a lemon followed by a tall glass of green goddess smoothie (page 218)

Crunchy cranberry quinola with fresh berries (page 102)

1–2 Brazil nuts

LUNCH

Collagen-building purple power slaw with citrus tahini dressing (page 122)

2 tablespoons of tummy-flattening ginger and caraway sauerkraut (page 124)

DINNER

Digestion-boosting basic garden salad (page 108)

Coconut and coriander red lentil dahl (page 179)

SNACKS

Green machine herbal cleanser (page 228)

Fresh fruit

Handful of pumpkin seeds

OPTIONAL EVENING TRYPTOPHAN-RICH SNACK TO BOOST SLEEP

Two gluten-free oatcakes with 1 teaspoon of almond or hazelnut butter or lemon and parsley hummus (page 145)

SUPPLEMENTS:

Vitamin B12

Probiotic capsule taken after dinner

DAY 4

BREAKFAST

Glass of warm water with the juice of half a lemon followed by a tall glass of green goddess smoothie (page 218)

Beauty mineral buckwheat porridge with blueberry chia jam (page 90)

1–2 Brazil nuts

LUNCH

Happy skin tabbouleh salad (page 112)

Immunity-boosting butternut squash, ginger and coconut soup (page 130)

Slice of omega-3 super bread (page 95)

DINNER

Raw courgetti with sun-dried tomato pesto (page 164)

Tummy-flattening ginger and caraway sauerkraut (page 124)

SNACKS

Green machine herbal cleanser (page 228)

Omega-3 kale crisps (page 238)

Fresh fruit

OPTIONAL EVENING TRYPTOPHAN-RICH SNACK TO BOOST SLEEP

Hormone-balancing chia and cinnamon thickshake (page 229)

SUPPLEMENTS

Vitamin B12

Probiotic capsule taken after dinner

DAY 5

BREAKFAST

Glass of warm water with the juice of half a lemon followed by a tall glass of green goddess smoothie (page 218)

Chocolate 'Nutella' overnight oats with strawberries and banana (page 84)

1–2 Brazil nuts

LUNCH

Rainbow glow bowl (page 114)

DINNER

Spicy pineapple salsa (page 146)

Loaded sweet potato nachos with zesty guacamole (page 163)

SNACKS

Rainbow berry blast (page 225)

Fresh fruit

Handful of pumpkin and sunflower seeds

OPTIONAL EVENING TRYPTOPHAN-RICH SNACK TO BOOST SLEEP

Sliced pear and a handful of sunflower seeds

SUPPLEMENTS

Vitamin B12

Probiotic capsule taken after dinner

DAY 6

BREAKFAST

Glass of warm water with the juice of half a lemon followed by a tall glass of green goddess smoothie (page 218)

Energy-boosting choco chia pudding (page 100)

1–2 Brazil nuts

LUNCH

Nori rainbow wraps with ginger sesame dressing (page 134)

DINNER

Digestion-boosting basic garden salad (page 108)

Quinoa colour dome with skin-brightening smoky sweet pepper and walnut dip (page 183)

SNACKS

Antioxidant matcha blueberry bombs (page 78)

Chocolate almond protein amazeballs (page 74)

Fresh fruit

Handful of walnuts or almonds

OPTIONAL EVENING TRYPTOPHAN-RICH SNACK TO BOOST SLEEP

Mashed banana with 1 teaspoon of almond or hazelnut butter and a sprinkle of ground cinnamon

SUPPLEMENTS

Vitamin B12

Probiotic capsule taken after dinner

DAY 7

BREAKFAST

Glass of warm water with the juice of half
a lemon followed by a tall glass of green
goddess smoothie (page 218)

Cinnamon spiced banana pancakes with
coconut milk yoghurt and blueberries (page
87)

1–2 Brazil nuts

LUNCH

Quinoa and hemp seed colour bowl
(page 111)

DINNER

Cucumber and carrot sticks with classic
tomato salsa (page 148)

Coconut curry with sweet potato noodles
(page 160)

SNACKS

A sweet treat or dessert of your choice!

OPTIONAL EVENING TRYPTOPHAN-RICH SNACK TO BOOST SLEEP

Slice of omega-3 super bread or toast (page
95) spread with mashed avocado

SUPPLEMENTS

Vitamin B12

Probiotic capsule taken after dinner

*Note: Please aim to buy organic and GM-free
ingredients as much as possible.*

RECOMMENDED KITCHEN TOOLS

I like to keep my meals and snacks simple, easy to clean up and fuss free, so I don't need a huge amount of different gadgets in my kitchen, but some are absolutely essential for creating the *Eat Yourself Beautiful* recipes and are definitely worth investing in.

BLENDER

To reap all the incredible beauty-boosting benefits of blended food like my daily staple, the green goddess smoothie, a decent blender will prove absolutely essential. It will be difficult to get the same results from the *Eat Yourself Beautiful* lifestyle without one. It could end up being one of the most valuable purchases you make for your health and will most likely even save you money on future doctor bills and prescriptions. Think of it as an investment in your well-being for life.

The Vitamix blender is one of the best on the market due to its industrial-grade strength. It's the one kitchen item that I absolutely couldn't live without, as I use it two or three times a day for my smoothies, soups, sauces, dressings and dips. It opened my eyes to a whole new world of delicious food and made the transition to a plant-based diet so much more easy and enjoyable. They are pricey, but if you can afford it, it's well worth the money.

The Nutribullet is another blender that gets excellent reviews and many of my friends who have one tell me how much they love it.

JUICER

I don't recommend that you make pure fruit juices, as the sugars wreak havoc on blood sugar levels when the fibre has been removed, but a green juice can be a refreshing alternative to smoothies and can be enjoyed as a light snack in the afternoon for an energy boost. One of the best juicers on the market is the Omega Vert, which is great for leafy greens and preserves their nutrients because it doesn't heat them up.

SALAD SPINNER

I use mine at least twice a day to wash various leafy greens. They're widely available, inexpensive and help you to stay on track with eating plenty of greens.

SPIRALISER

I bought a spiraliser a year or two ago because I was keen to try raw courgette spaghetti. It turned out to be a worthwhile investment because I use it about four times a week as it's so versatile. I use it to spiralise sweet potatoes, cucumbers, carrots and apples to add taste, texture and versatility to raw and cooked dishes. A vegetable peeler can also achieve a similar result.

DEHYDRATOR

This is optional, as much of what is done in a dehydrator can also be done using an oven at a very low heat. I prefer to concentrate on fresh, water-rich foods, but I was given an Excalibur dehydrator as a present a few years ago and it's great for making kale crisps and raw flax crackers. It's a box with shelves and a fan at the back, which slowly warms and dries out food and preserves the vital nutrients and enzymes that would otherwise be lost in cooking.

TABLESPOONS AND TEASPOONS

I use measuring spoons for the smaller ingredients in my recipes, so the correct size spoon is important.

SHARP KNIVES

I use a serrated knife to chop up tougher fruits and veggies, like pineapple, raw squash and sweet potato. Sharp knives get prep work done quicker and you actually have a lower chance of cutting your fingers because food is less likely to slip out from under them, which can happen with blunt knives.

MUSLIN CLOTH OR CHEESECLOTH

A muslin cloth or cheesecloth is handy for straining nut milk and for draining excess liquid when making nut and seed cheeses.

STORE CUPBOARD STAPLES

Please see the Shopping List section of my website, www.RosannaDavisonNutrition.com, for my recommended list of pantry staples.

EATING OUT AND TRAVELLING

For my tips on how to stick to the *Eat Yourself Beautiful* eating plan when in restaurants and while travelling, see the posts on my website, www.RosannaDavisonNutrition.com.

BREAKFAST

The *Eat Yourself Beautiful* programme will help to transform your health and beauty best when you drink a cup of warm water with lemon or lime juice upon waking, followed by a large, cold glass of the green goddess smoothie (page 218). Those of you who are used to eating a heavier breakfast can then choose from one of the breakfast options in this chapter. You may find that over time you will be satisfied with just the smoothie. It all depends on your own metabolism, age, gender and activity levels, so listen to your body and get used to receiving its hunger and thirst signals.

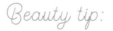

Beauty tip:

CINNAMON IS A TRUE BEAUTY SPICE.
IT HELPS TO REGULATE PESKY
SUGAR CRAVINGS AND STABILISE
BLOOD SUGAR LEVELS DUE TO ITS
CHROMIUM CONTENT. IT ALSO FIGHTS
FUNGAL INFECTIONS, BOOSTS BLOOD
CIRCULATION AND IS A RICH SOURCE
OF MINERALS AND ANTIOXIDANTS.

CHOCOLATE ALMOND PROTEIN AMAZEBALLS

Makes 11–12 balls

4 scoops of chocolate flavour Sunwarrior raw vegan protein powder (the vanilla flavour works too)

6 tbsp raw unsalted smooth almond butter (the drippier, the better!)

4 tbsp raw cacao powder

4 tbsp sesame seeds

3 ¹/₂–4 tbsp liquid sweetener, such as pure organic maple syrup, organic coconut nectar or raw local honey (if not vegan)

2 tsp ground cinnamon

2 tsp vanilla extract

10 tbsp unsweetened almond milk

TO COAT:

3–4 tbsp cacao powder

3–4 tbsp unsweetened desiccated coconut

These balls of tasty, nutritious goodness are the perfect way to restore energy levels and repair torn muscle fibres after a workout. I often pop a couple into a small airtight container to enjoy after a weights session or a Pilates class. I use raw vegan protein powder and include antioxidant-rich raw cacao to help fight the damaging free radicals that we all produce through strenuous exercise, while the raw almond butter gives you a boost of fibre and skin-friendly fats, vitamin E and beauty minerals. Guilt-free snacking at its best!

1　Place the protein powder, almond butter, cacao powder, sesame seeds, liquid sweetener, cinnamon and vanilla extract in a large mixing bowl. Add the almond milk one tablespoon at a time, mixing all the ingredients with your hands until the 'dough' begins to stick together but doesn't get too wet. Roll the mixture into 11 or 12 balls in the palms of your hands until well rounded and smooth.

2　Put the cacao powder and desiccated coconut in two separate bowls. Roll the balls around in one or the other until well coated.

3　Keep chilled in the fridge until ready to serve. These can be stored in an airtight container in the fridge for up to three days.

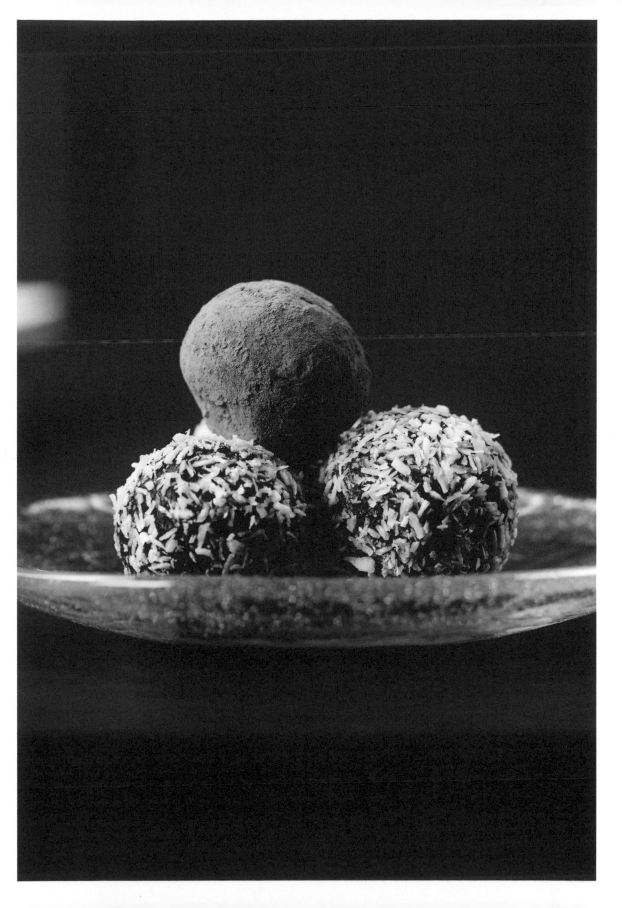

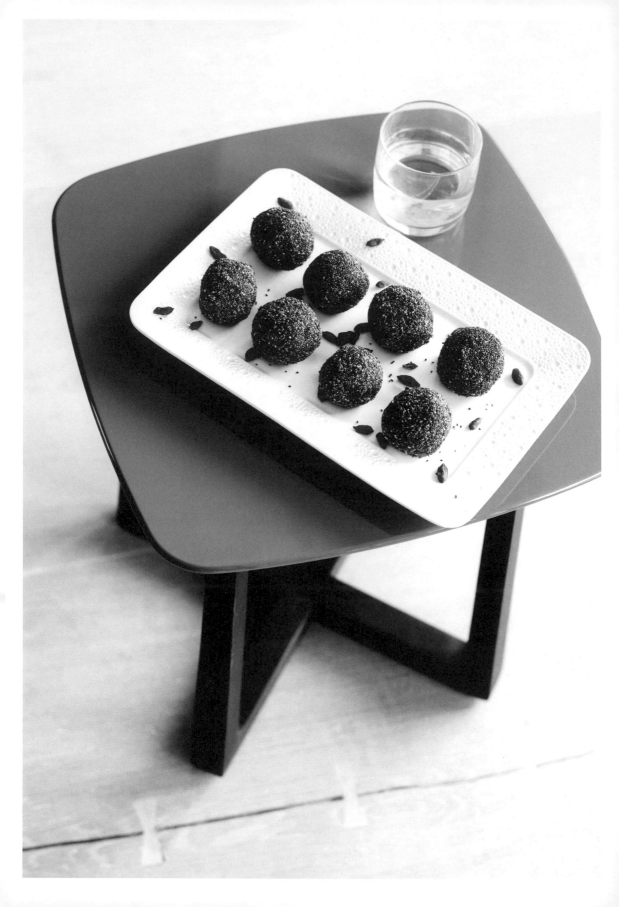

VANILLA, CASHEW AND GOJI PROTEIN AMAZEBALLS

Makes 11–12 balls

4 scoops of vanilla flavour Sunwarrior raw vegan protein powder

6 tbsp raw cashew butter

3 $\frac{1}{2}$–4 tbsp liquid sweetener, such as pure organic maple syrup, organic coconut nectar or raw local honey (if not vegan)

2 tbsp dried goji berries

2 tsp ground cinnamon

2 tsp vanilla extract

10 tbsp unsweetened almond milk

4 tbsp whole chia seeds, to coat

These are a variation on the chocolate almond protein amaze-balls on page 74 for those who prefer vanilla to chocolate! They're just as simple, nutritious and tasty, plus the goji berries and chia seeds add a heap of antioxidants, minerals, omega-3 fats and fibre. I love to leave them in the fridge to chill for an hour to let the berries get really hard and crunchy.

1   Place the protein powder, cashew butter, liquid sweetener, goji berries, cinnamon and vanilla extract in a large mixing bowl. Add the almond milk one tablespoon at a time, mixing all the ingredients with your hands until the 'dough' begins to stick together but doesn't get too wet. Roll the mixture into 11 or 12 balls in the palms of your hands until well rounded and smooth.

2   Place the chia seeds in a separate small bowl. Roll the balls around in them until well coated.

3   Keep chilled in the fridge until ready to serve. These can be stored in an airtight container in the fridge for up to three days.

ANTIOXIDANT MATCHA BLUEBERRY BOMBS

Makes 8 balls

150g Medjool dates, pitted

16 blueberries

$\frac{1}{2}$ tsp vanilla seeds or pure vanilla extract

60g raw unsalted almond butter

2 heaped tbsp raw cacao powder

2 tbsp raw hulled hemp seeds

1 tbsp pure organic maple syrup or coconut nectar

2 heaped tbsp matcha green tea powder

These bright green balls are an ideal breakfast or snack for those who love their daily caffeine fix but are looking for an alternative to coffee. Matcha tea is a unique Japanese green tea powder. What makes it so special is its rich content of wrinkle-fighting antioxidants, beauty nutrients, tummy-flattening fibre and chlorophyll for cleansed, oxygenated blood. While still caffeinated, it provides a gentler and more sustained lift than the instant hit of coffee, which can make many of us feel anxious and jittery. It also contains an amino acid called L-theanine, which has a calming effect. These raw food 'bombs' pack a serious antioxidant punch to fight the signs of ageing, as they're packed with whole foods, omega-3 fats, fibre, raw cacao powder, blueberries and matcha green tea powder.

1   Soak the dates in warm water for 15–20 minutes to soften them.
2   Rinse the blueberries and place them in a small bowl with the vanilla. Mash the berries with a fork to gently crush them and allow their juices to mix with the vanilla.
3   Places the dates, almond butter, cacao powder, hemp seeds and maple syrup in a blender and combine until a thick 'dough' is formed. You may need to add a splash of water to help it all blend together. Roll the date and almond butter mixture into eight balls between the palms of your hands.
4   Cut each ball evenly in half. Use your thumb to make a small indent on the inside of each half and fill with $\frac{1}{2}$ teaspoon of the blueberry mixture. Put the halves back together, pressing firmly to ensure they don't break apart.
5   Place the matcha green tea powder in a bowl and roll each ball around in it until they're fully coated.
6   Keep the balls chilled in the fridge until ready to serve. Store in an airtight container in the fridge for up to three days.

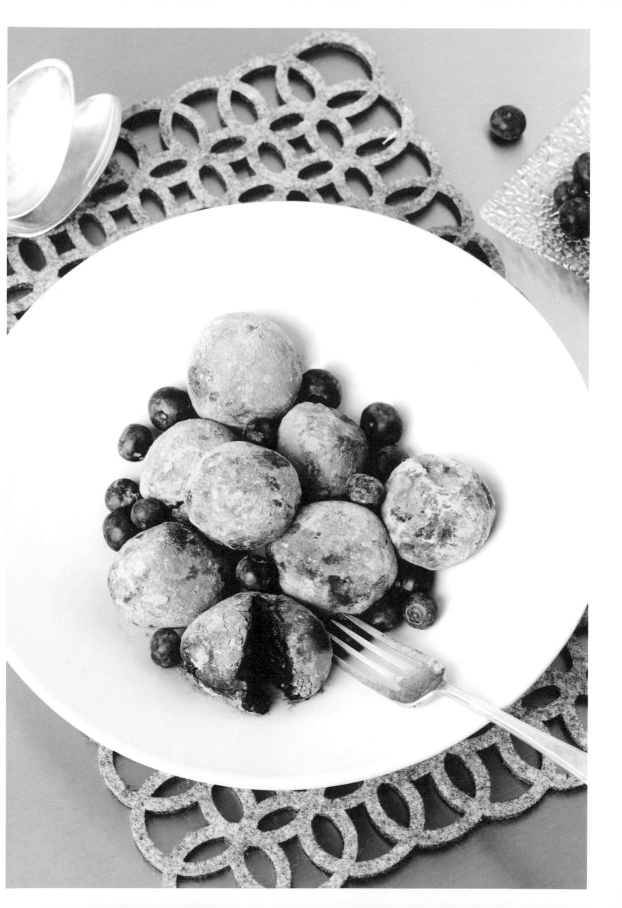

CHIA OAT PARFAIT WITH RASPBERRY CHIA JAM

Serves 2

FOR THE CHIA OAT PARFAIT:

60g gluten-free rolled oats

2 ¹/₂ tbsp chia seeds

1 tsp ground cinnamon

1 tsp vanilla extract

500ml dairy-free milk (I use either unsweetened almond or low-fat coconut milk)

selection of fresh fruit – berries, chopped bananas, peaches, figs and kiwi all work well

FOR THE RASPBERRY CHIA JAM:

1 tbsp pure maple syrup

250g frozen raspberries

juice of ¹/₂ lemon

2 tbsp chia seeds

This overnight parfait is perfect to grab from the fridge in the morning for a tasty weekday breakfast when you're in a hurry. The combined chia and oats keep you feeling full for hours, while the chia jam is deceptively simple to make and adds a colourful burst of skin-boosting antioxidants.

1   To make the raspberry chia jam, heat the maple syrup in a saucepan over a medium heat until it begins to gently bubble. Add the frozen raspberries and lemon juice, stirring well, and simmer until the berries begin to break down and liquefy. Taste at this point and add a little more maple syrup if you prefer it sweeter, though I like it quite tart. Add the chia seeds and stir well for 60 seconds. Turn off the heat and continue to stir until the chia seeds begin to absorb the liquid from the raspberries and swell up. Pour the jam into a container or jar and set in the fridge for 1 hour.

2   To make the parfait, mix together the oats, chia seeds, cinnamon, vanilla extract and plant milk in a bowl.

3   Now for the fun part! Layer up the parfait in a glass jar, starting with a layer of the oats, followed by a layer of raspberry chia jam, until you have filled the jar almost to the top. Screw the lid on top and leave in the fridge overnight to let the flavours blend together.

4   In the morning, add your fresh fruit to the top of the jar, grab a spoon and enjoy! It's as simple as that.

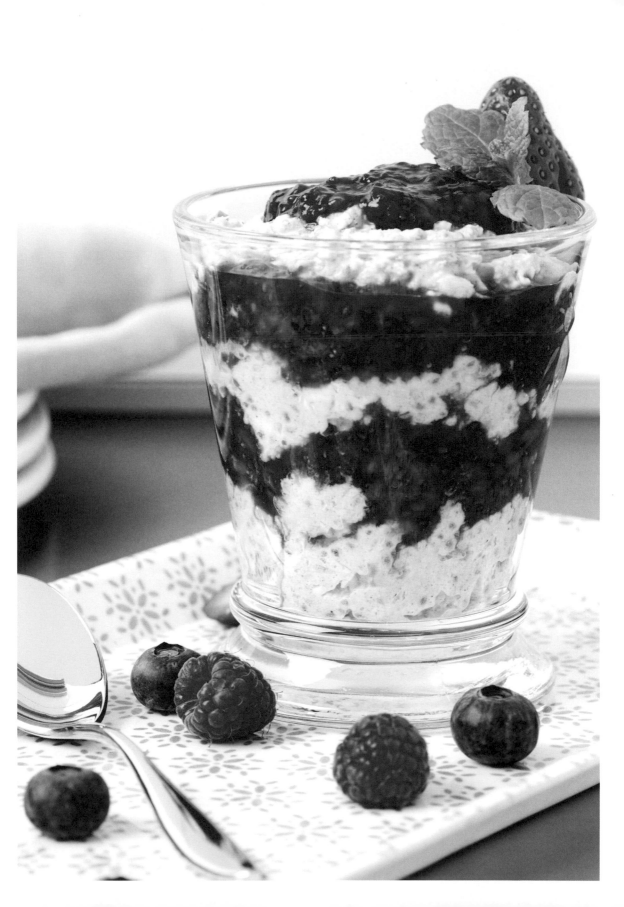

CREAMY BERRY AND COCONUT QUINOA PORRIDGE

Serves 2

170g quinoa

500ml low-fat coconut milk
(I use the type from a carton
rather than the thick coconut
milk in a tin)

1 tbsp pure maple syrup or
honey (optional)

1 tsp ground cinnamon

1 tsp vanilla extract

handful of fresh mixed
berries (I love blueberries and
raspberries in this dish)

2 tbsp unsweetened shredded
or desiccated coconut

2 tbsp chopped pecans,
lightly toasted

It's hard to beat a warm, satisfying breakfast on a chilly morning, although this creamy coconut quinoa porridge is a great evening snack too. Since quinoa is a complete protein, containing all eight essential amino acids plus fibre and a multitude of minerals, it's a super-nourishing alternative to classic oatmeal. It will absorb any flavour, but my favourite is coconut and vanilla with fresh berries, which works so well with the sweet, nutty taste of toasted pecans.

1 Rinse the quinoa well in a sieve under cold running water.
2 In a saucepan, heat up the coconut milk over a medium heat until it's nearly at boiling point. Pour the quinoa into the milk, stir it well and cover partly with a lid. Reduce the heat to a gentle simmer and cook for 10–12 minutes, until the quinoa seeds begin to open up. Remove the lid for the final 3 minutes of the cooking time to allow the remaining liquid to evaporate. Quinoa should be light and fluffy, so take care not to let it burn.
3 Mix in the sweetener (if using), cinnamon and vanilla with a fork to fluff up the quinoa.
4 Spoon the quinoa porridge into two serving bowls. Top with the berries, coconut, toasted pecans and another pinch of ground cinnamon.

NUTTY BANANA FITNESS FLAPJACKS

Makes about 9 flapjacks

1 tsp coconut oil, for greasing

2 large, ripe bananas

150g gluten-free rolled oats

40g dried organic apricots, chopped

40g chopped nuts, such as walnuts, hazelnuts, almonds or pecans

2 tbsp seeds, such as flax, sunflower or pumpkin

1 tsp vanilla extract

1/2 tsp ground cinnamon

pinch of ground nutmeg

This is one of the easiest, quickest, healthiest and most versatile breakfasts, snacks and desserts there is. A batch can be whipped up in about 40 minutes, start to finish. They are perfect for lunch boxes, as an elevenses snack or a post-school/college/work/gym filler until dinner. They also satisfy that mid-afternoon energy slump, as the dried apricots add a pop of high-fibre sweetness without compromising your healthy eating plan. The bananas alone take the place of sugar, fat and eggs – a magic ingredient! Apricots are also a good source of iron to help support energy levels and transport oxygen to every cell in your body.

1   Preheat the oven to 190°C. Lightly grease a 23cm x 23cm square baking tin with coconut oil.

2   Peel the bananas and put them in a mixing bowl. Mash very thoroughly until no large chunks remain and they're almost liquid. Stir in the oats, apricots, nuts, seeds, vanilla and cinnamon and mix well to combine.

3   Pat the thick mixture evenly into the baking pan. Dust a little ground nutmeg lightly across the top.

4   Bake for about 30 minutes, until the edges are just beginning to get brown and crispy.

5   Place the baking tin on a wire rack to cool. When the pan is mostly cool, cut the flapjacks into bars. Store in an airtight container in the fridge for up to three days.

CHOCOLATE 'NUTELLA' OVERNIGHT OATS WITH STRAWBERRIES AND BANANA

Serves 2

6 heaped tbsp gluten-free oats

2 tbsp chia seeds

2 tsp ground cinnamon

500ml unsweetened almond milk

2 heaped tbsp healthy homemade 'Nutella' (page 86)

chopped bananas, to serve

chopped fresh strawberries, to serve

I still dream of the great chunks of fresh bread slathered with Nutella that I ate for breakfast as a child whenever I stayed with my cousins in their Italian home. It felt like the ultimate indulgence as I licked the gooey chocolate spread from my lips and fingertips. Nutella for breakfast is still possible on the *Eat Yourself Beautiful* programme, as this healthy breakfast option proves. Free from refined sugar but oozing with flavour for every chocoholic out there, this is such a simple and quick breakfast to whip up, plus kids adore it too.

1 Mix together the oats, chia seeds and cinnamon in a bowl, then divide between two jars or bowls and pour the almond milk over them. I like to use glass jars for overnight oats, as they are easy to bring to work, college or school, but a glass tumbler or normal cereal bowl work too.

2 Place 1 tablespoon of the homemade 'Nutella' on top of each portion. Cover and leave in the fridge overnight.

3 In the morning, stir the 'Nutella' into the oats. Top with freshly chopped bananas and strawberries.

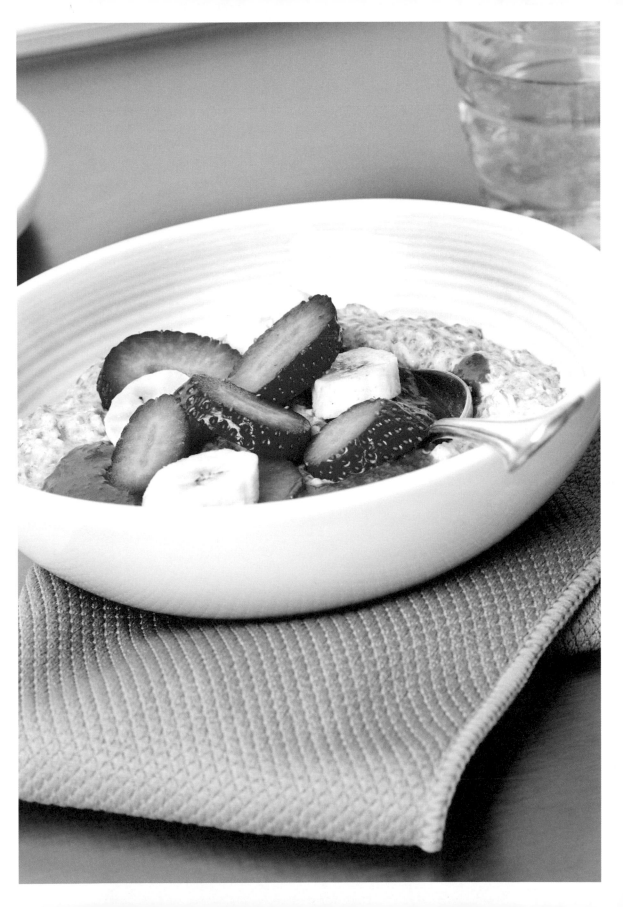

HEALTHY HOMEMADE 'NUTELLA'

Makes 1 small jar

150g roasted whole hazelnuts

150g pitted dates, chopped

120ml cold water

3 heaped tbsp organic raw cacao powder

2 tbsp pure organic maple syrup

1 tsp vanilla extract

1 Soak the hazelnuts in a small bowl of cold water for 6–8 hours. Soak the dates in a separate small bowl of warm water for 15–20 minutes to soften them.

2 Drain the nuts and dates and place them in your blender or food processor along with the cold water, cacao powder, maple syrup and vanilla extract. Blend together until smooth and creamy. Add a little extra water to help it blend if necessary.

3 Transfer to a jar and store in the fridge, covered, for up to four days.

CINNAMON SPICED BANANA PANCAKES WITH COCONUT MILK YOGHURT AND BLUEBERRIES

Makes 6 pancakes

1 ripe banana, peeled

450ml unsweetened almond milk

1 tsp ground cinnamon

1 tsp vanilla extract

$\frac{1}{2}$ tsp ground nutmeg

5 drops of liquid stevia

150g buckwheat flour

pinch of Himalayan pink rock salt

1 tbsp coconut oil

coconut milk yoghurt, to serve

handful of blueberries, to serve

Banana and cinnamon are a classic combination, warmed up by the fragrant flavour of the nutmeg. These pancakes are really filling yet easy to digest, as buckwheat is a seed rather than a grain and is naturally gluten free. The blueberries add a healthy dose of antioxidants, while the creamy coconut milk yoghurt melts decadently over the hot pancakes.

1   Put the banana, almond milk, cinnamon, vanilla, nutmeg and stevia in a blender and whizz until smooth.

2   Place the flour and a pinch of salt in a large mixing bowl. Make a well in the middle and slowly stir in the wet mixture until a smooth batter is formed.

3   Heat the coconut oil in a large frying pan over a medium heat until it bubbles. Pour in 2 tablespoons of the batter and cook until the edges begin to lift. Gently flip the pancake over and cook on the other side until golden brown.

4   Transfer the pancakes to a serving plate with a dollop of coconut milk yoghurt and some blueberries. Serve hot.

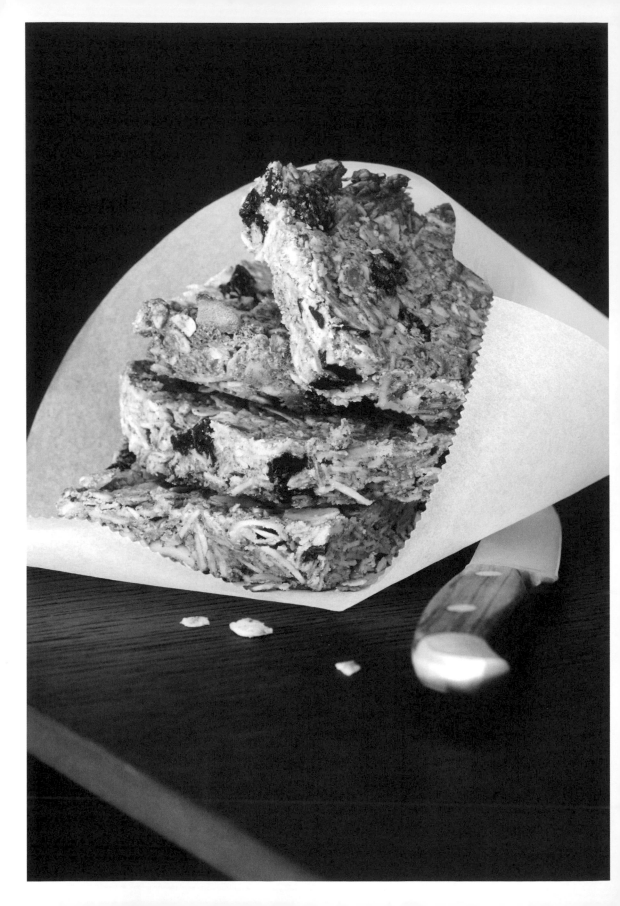

CHERRY COCONUT RECOVERY BARS

Makes 16 bars

150g gluten-free rolled oats

100g sliced almonds

80g unsweetened dried tart cherries

50g unsweetened coconut flakes

155g pure organic maple syrup or coconut nectar

125g raw unsalted almond butter

1 tbsp coconut oil, plus extra for greasing

1 tsp pure vanilla extract

1/2 tsp ground cinnamon

As the substantial and ever-increasing body of scientific research attests, tart cherries are abundant in anti-inflammatory and health-protective phytonutrients, which help to ease post-workout muscle pain and stiff joints and enhance our sleep. I also never seem to get bored of easy, healthy and delicious granola bars as a breakfast or post-exercise snack, and the pop of sweet cherry alongside toasted almonds and coconut is a divine combination. I make a big batch at the start of the week with the intention of going through them slowly, but that never seems to happen as friends and family love to munch on them whenever they call over for a cup of tea.

1 Preheat the oven to 190°C. Lightly grease a large baking tray with coconut oil.

2 Place the oats, almonds, cherries and coconut flakes in a large mixing bowl and combine well. Pour the mixture onto the baking tray and lightly toast in the oven for 10–12 minutes, stirring after 5 minutes. Remove from the oven and place it back in the mixing bowl.

3 Meanwhile, in a small saucepan set over a medium heat, warm the maple syrup, almond butter, coconut oil, vanilla and cinnamon until the oil is melted. Mix well.

4 Add the wet ingredients to the oats and stir until well combined. Pour the mixture back onto the baking tray. Even it out and press down firmly to ensure the ingredients all stick together.

5 Bake for 10–15 minutes, until firm to the touch. Transfer to a wire cooling rack and allow the bars to cool fo 10 minutes before cutting into bars. Store the bars in an airtight container in the fridge for up to four days.

BEAUTY MINERAL BUCK-WHEAT PORRIDGE WITH BLUEBERRY CHIA JAM

Serves 3–4

325g raw buckwheat groats

1 litre cold water

300ml unsweetened almond milk

2 tbsp chia seeds

1 heaped tsp ground cinnamon

1 tsp vanilla extract

3–4 tbsp pure organic maple syrup, coconut nectar or raw honey (optional)

handful of fresh blueberries, to serve

FOR THE BLUEBERRY CHIA JAM:

1 tbsp pure maple syrup

250g frozen blueberries

juice of ½ lemon

2 tbsp chia seeds

We're all familiar with regular oat porridge, but raw buckwheat porridge clocks in quite a bit higher in the nutrition stakes. Even better, there's absolutely no cooking needed! This superfood breakfast combines naturally gluten-free buckwheat groats with chia seeds and blueberries for a meal that's jam-packed with protein, calcium, magnesium and essential omega-3 fats for smooth skin and a sharp mind.

1   First soak the groats in a bowl with 1 litre of cold water for 1–2 hours. Once soaked, rinse well in a sieve or strainer.

2   To make the blueberry chia jam, heat the maple syrup in a saucepan over a medium heat until it begins to gently bubble. Add the frozen blueberries and lemon juice, stirring well, and simmer until the berries begin to break down and liquefy. Taste at this point and add a little more maple syrup if you prefer it sweeter, though I like it quite tart. Add the chia seeds and stir well for 30–60 seconds. Turn off the heat and continue to stir until the chia seeds begin to absorb the liquid from the blueberries and swell up. Pour the jam into a container or jar and set in the fridge for 1 hour.

3   Put the soaked groats in a blender or food processor with the almond milk, chia seeds, cinnamon and vanilla and blend until smooth. Taste and add the sweetener if required.

4   Serve in bowls topped with a dollop of blueberry chia jam and some fresh blueberries.

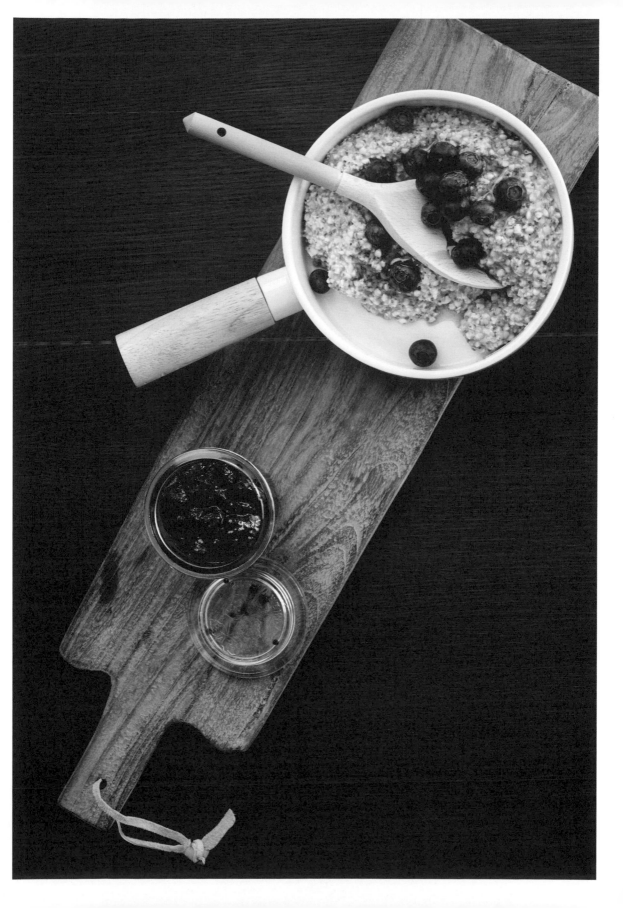

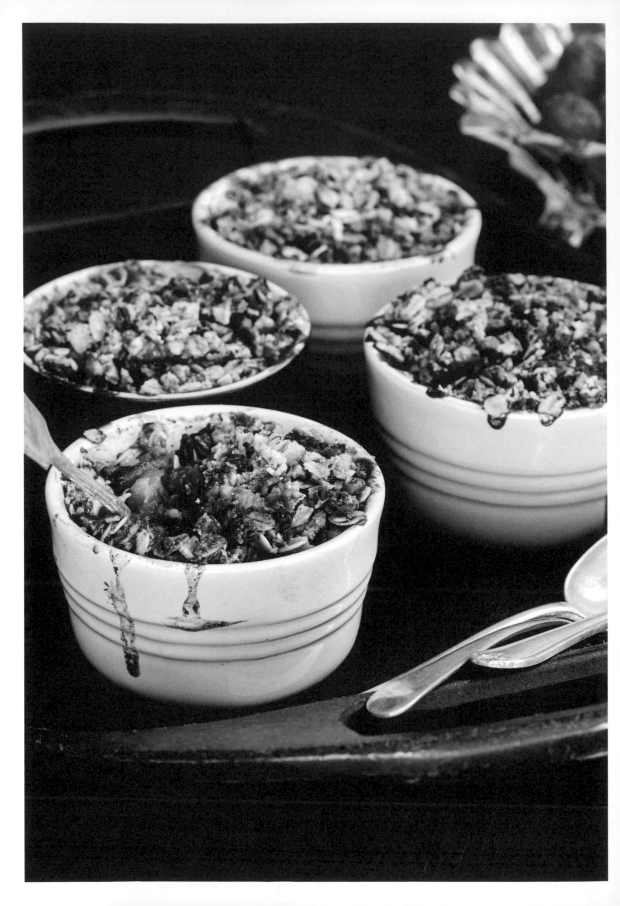

RUSTIC SPICED PEAR AND RASPBERRY BREAKFAST CRUMBLE

Serves 4

coconut oil, for greasing

125g fresh raspberries

4 medium pears, cored and cut into bite-sized chunks

3 tbsp freshly squeezed lemon juice

1 tbsp organic coconut palm sugar, xylitol or pure organic maple syrup

1 heaped tsp ground cinnamon

1 tsp vanilla extract

FOR THE CRUMBLE TOPPING:

110g gluten-free rolled oats

80g pecan nuts, chopped

20g ground almonds

4 tbsp pure organic maple syrup or coconut palm nectar (optional)

3 tbsp coconut oil, melted

pinch of ground cinnamon

This is a deceptively simple and warming breakfast that could also pass for a satisfying dessert. The warming flavours of pear and cinnamon are sharpened by the raspberries, which give it a beautiful summery colour. The soft fruits complement the crisp oatmeal perfectly and the dish is a great source of fibre, which cleanses the digestive system for glowing good health.

1   Preheat the oven to 180°C. Lightly grease four ramekins with coconut oil.
2   Mix together the raspberries, pears, lemon juice, sweetener, cinnamon and vanilla extract in a bowl. Divide between the ramekins, making sure the top is flat and even.
3   In a separate bowl, combine the oats, pecans, ground almonds, sweetener and coconut oil. Spread the oats in a layer across the fruit in the ramekins and sprinkle with a pinch of cinnamon.
4   Bake in the oven for about 40 minutes, until the pears are tender and the topping is crispy. Allow to cool slightly before serving.

COSY APPLE CRUMBLE BAKED OATMEAL

Serves 2

75g gluten-free oats

2 tbsp mixed seeds, such as sunflower, pumpkin and flaxseed

1 tbsp organic raisins

2 tsp organic coconut palm sugar, organic maple syrup, stevia or xylitol

2 tsp ground cinnamon, plus extra for sprinkling

1/2 tsp ground nutmeg

500ml unsweetened almond milk

1 medium apple

2 tbsp raw almond butter, to drizzle

There are few better taste combinations than baked apple with cinnamon. It conjures up wonderful childhood memories of my grandmother's home cooking and the warmth of her country kitchen in autumn, when ripe apples from the farm's own orchard would be harvested and baked into tarts and crumbles. This easy breakfast recipe for baked apple with cinnamon brings together those classic cosy flavours and will make your home smell of apple crumble. It only takes 5 minutes to prepare and 15–20 minutes to bake, so it's perfect for popping into the oven while you get ready for the day before sitting down to a wholesome, filling breakfast. I use organic coconut palm sugar to sweeten it slightly, which gives it a gorgeous butterscotch taste. Coconut palm sugar is unrefined and made from the nectar of coconut palm blossoms. If you can't find it, a drizzle of good-quality maple syrup, raw honey (if you're not vegan) or a teaspoon of a plant-based sweetener like stevia or xylitol would also add a little bit of sweetness.

1 Preheat the oven to 190°C.

2 Mix the oats, seeds, raisins, your choice of sweetener, cinnamon and nutmeg in a large bowl and pour over the almond milk. Grate or finely chop the apple, reserving two slices for garnish, and mix into the oatmeal, stirring well to combine everything.

3 Transfer the oatmeal to two oven-safe bowls and sprinkle a little extra cinnamon on top of each one. Bake for 15–20 minutes, until the top is brown and crisp.

4 Drizzle each bowl with 1 tablespoon of almond butter, add a slice of fresh apple and serve warm.

OMEGA-3 SUPER BREAD

Makes 1 loaf

1 tsp coconut oil, for greasing

145g whole raw unsalted almonds

130g pumpkin seeds

160g brown rice flour

85g whole flaxseeds

70g sunflower seeds

3 heaped tbsp psyllium husk powder

2 tbsp chia seeds

pinch of Himalayan pink rock salt

500ml cold water

Make a loaf or two of this super bread at the beginning of the week and it should last for a few days' worth of meals and snacks.

1   Put the almonds and pumpkin seeds in a food processor or blender and blend until a flour forms. Place this flour into a bowl and combine with the rice flour, flaxseeds, sunflower seeds, psyllium husk powder, chia seeds and a pinch of salt. Stir the mixture as you pour in the cold water.
2   Allow to sit for 1 hour to let the dry ingredients absorb the liquid and to let the 'dough' firm up.
3   Once it's really firm, preheat the oven to 190°C. Lightly grease a loaf tin with coconut oil.
4   Transfer the 'dough' to the greased loaf tin and press it down well with the back of a spoon.
5   Bake for 40-50 minutes, until the top is turning brown and a knife inserted into the middle comes out clean, without any mixture sticking to it.
6   Turn the bread out of the tin and enjoy while warm, or it can be kept in the fridge for two or three days in a sealed container and it toasts well. It can also be sliced and frozen.

OMEGA-3 SUPER TOAST WITH SMASHED CHILLI-LIME AVOCADO

Serves 2

1 ripe avocado

juice of 1 lime

$^1/_2$ tsp chilli flakes

Himalayan pink rock salt and freshly ground black pepper

a few slices of omega-3 super bread (page 95)

The creamy, wholesome simplicity of avocado on toast is seriously difficult to beat with its melt-in-the-mouth buttery texture against warm, crunchy toast. While it makes a great snack or light meal served with a bowl of soup, this avocado toast is the perfect breakfast as it's rich in essential fats, fibre, plant protein and beauty vitamins and minerals. For a sweet variation, try it with homemade almond butter and the raspberry chia jam on page 80.

1   Cut the avocado in half lengthways and remove the stone. Scoop the flesh into a bowl and add the lime juice, chilli flakes and seasoning. Mash it all together until smooth.
2   Spread thickly on the toasted omega-3 super bread and enjoy straightaway.

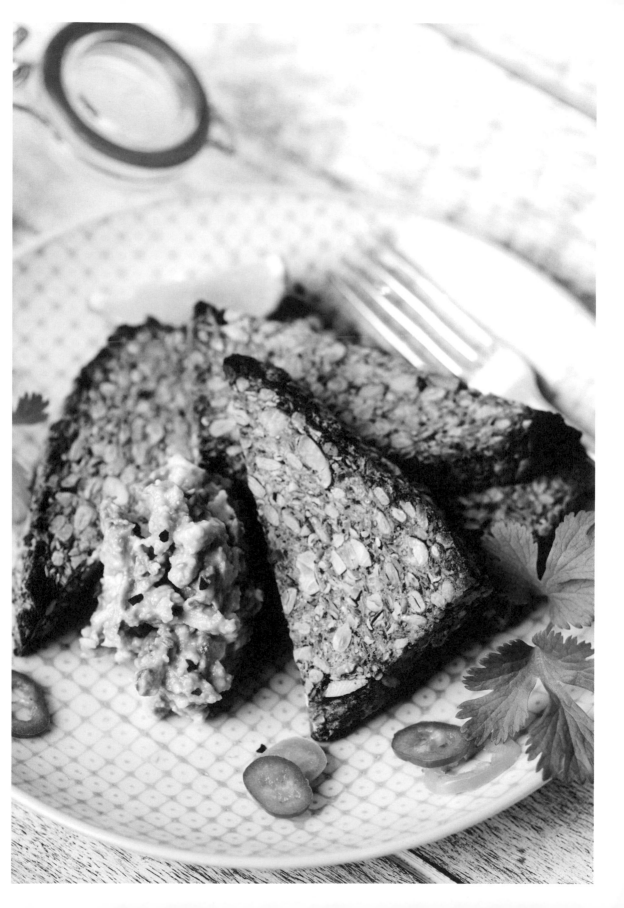

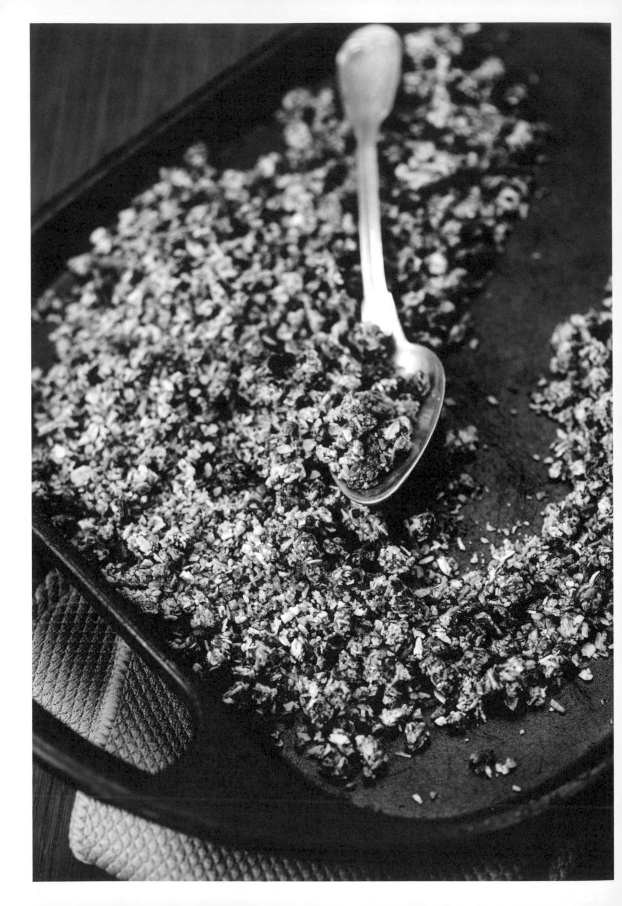

CHEWY COCONUT DATE GRANOLA

Serves 2–3

75g dates, pitted and chopped

40g gluten-free oats

40g unsweetened desiccated coconut

4–5 drops pure liquid stevia for sweetness (optional)

1 tsp ground cinnamon

1 tsp vanilla extract

splash of almond or coconut milk, if needed

This makes a good alternative to crunchy granola and doesn't contain any added oils. The dates are a natural sweetener and make it really chewy, which works well with the oats and coconut. I like to sprinkle it over smoothies and porridge or just munch on handfuls of it as an anytime snack.

1. Soak the dates in a small bowl of warm water for 15–20 minutes to soften them. Drain well.
2. Preheat the oven to 210°C. Lightly grease a baking tray with coconut oil.
3. Put all the ingredients into a blender or food processor and whizz together until it becomes dough-like. Add a little almond or coconut milk to help it blend if needed.
4. Pour out onto the greased baking tray and separate the mixture into granola-sized bits so it's not all in one lump. I find it easiest to do this with my hands.
5. Bake in the oven for 15–20 minutes, until browned. Once out of the oven, allow the granola to cool and become crispy. The granola is best eaten on the day it's made, but can be stored for one or two days in an airtight container.

ENERGY-BOOSTING CHOCO CHIA PUDDING

Serves 3–4

4 heaped tbsp chia seeds

250ml cold water

500ml unsweetened almond milk

2 Medjool dates, pitted

3 tbsp raw cacao powder

2 tbsp ground flaxseed

2 tbsp organic coconut palm nectar or pure organic maple syrup (optional)

2 tsp ground cinnamon

mixed berries, to serve

chopped raw almonds, to serve

Women have a slightly higher requirement for iron due to the monthly menstrual cycle, and anaemia is a rather common condition amongst my female clients. With symptoms that include fatigue, dizziness and breathlessness, anaemia can be incredibly frustrating for sufferers trying to lead a normal life. I'm very careful to keep my iron levels high with plenty of green veggies, pulses and legumes, but this choco chia pudding is also a great source of iron to boost everyday energy levels, especially for active types. Plus it tastes delicious!

1   Soak the chia seeds in the cold water for 10 minutes to allow them to swell up.
2   Add the expanded chia seeds to the unsweetened almond milk and mix together well. Place in the fridge for 15 minutes to set.
3   In a food processor or blender, blend the dates, cacao powder, ground flaxseed, the sweetener (if using) and the cinnamon. Add the almond milk and chia seed mixture and blend together well.
4   Transfer to serving bowls and top with the mixed berries and chopped raw almonds.

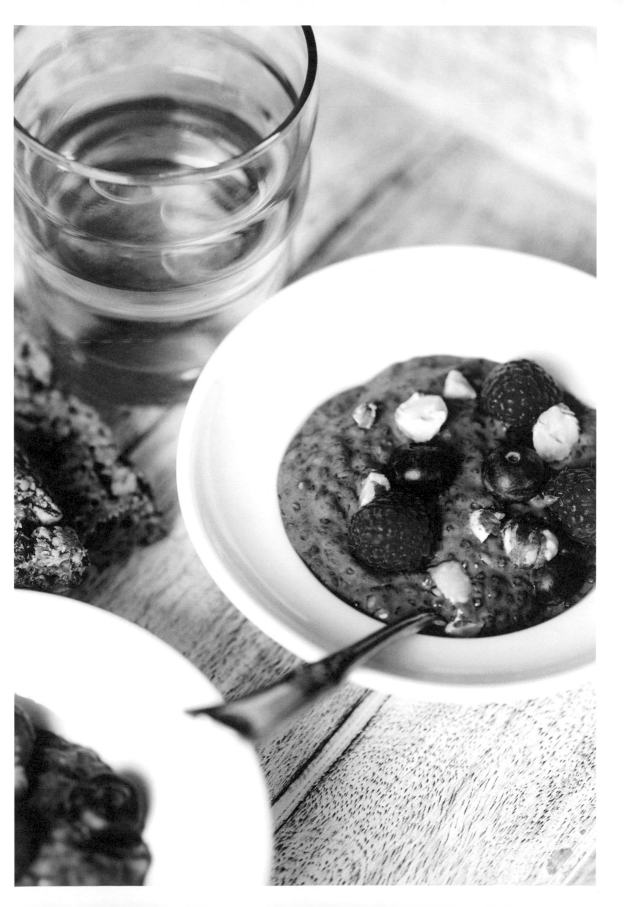

CRUNCHY CRANBERRY QUINOLA

Serves 2–3

1 tsp coconut oil, for greasing

1 medium, ripe banana, mashed well

1 tbsp tahini

1 tbsp organic pure maple syrup or coconut palm nectar

1 tsp vanilla extract

150g quinoa flakes

110g raw unsalted whole almonds, chopped

40g chopped walnuts

30g pumpkin seeds

20g desiccated coconut

2 tbsp sunflower seeds

2 tbsp ground flaxseed

2 tsp ground cinnamon

25g dried unsweetened cranberries

2 tbsp goji berries

2 tbsp whole flaxseeds

I don't think I know anybody who doesn't like crunchy granola. It's so versatile and is delicious sprinkled on smoothies, fruit salads, porridge, chia puddings or just on its own drenched in ice-cold almond milk as a breakfast or snack. But rather than buying a commercial brand full of refined sugar and unhealthy fats, this easy homemade version uses wholesome, high-fibre ingredients, tahini instead of oil and it even replaces oats with quinoa flakes for a better nutritional boost. The cranberries and goji berries add a pleasant pop of sweetness.

1   Preheat the oven to 125°C. Lightly grease a baking tray with coconut oil.
2   Mix the banana, tahini, maple syrup and vanilla extract in a large bowl until well combined. Add the quinoa flakes, almonds, walnuts, pumpkin seeds, coconut, sunflower seeds, ground flaxseed and cinnamon and stir until it stick together in clumps.
3   Spread the mixture evenly across the greased baking tray. Place in the oven and gently toast for 45 minutes, giving it a mix every 15 minutes.
4   Remove from the oven when it's golden brown and mix in the cranberries, goji berries and whole flaxseeds. Allow the granola to cool completely before storing in an airtight container in the fridge for up to three days.

CHEWY CRANBERRY GINGER ENERGY BARS

Makes 12 bars

110g pitted dates

coconut oil, for greasing

115g rolled oats

30g dried unsweetened cranberries

30g pumpkin seeds

30g raw sunflower seeds

4 heaped tbsp chia seeds

1 tbsp finely chopped fresh ginger

1 tsp ground cinnamon

1 tsp vanilla extract

250ml water

These energy bars make a great breakfast and anytime snack as they're loaded with fibre, protein, essential fats, vitamins and minerals. I love to munch on one as a pick-me-up after a strenuous Pilates class or sweaty run as they're so filling and loaded with goodness. Rather than using sugar, I have sweetened these bars naturally with date paste. I've also added a little fresh ginger, which boosts the immune system and improves digestion to keep you healthy and energised all year long.

1   Soak the dates in a small bowl of warm water for 15–20 minutes to soften them. Drain well.
2   Preheat the oven to 190°C. Lightly grease a large baking tray with coconut oil.
3   Pour the oats into a blender and process until they become a fine flour. Transfer to a large mixing bowl and add the cranberries, pumpkin seeds, sunflower seeds, chia seeds, ginger, cinnamon and vanilla.
4   Add the soaked dates to the blender with 250ml water and blend to a smooth paste. Pour the date paste into the bowl of dry ingredients and mix together well. Pour the mixture into the greased baking tray and use a spatula to even it out.
5   Bake for about 25 minutes, until golden brown. Remove from the oven and transfer to a cooling rack. Allow to cool for 10 minutes before cutting into bars. Store the bars in an airtight container for up to four days.

SWEET COCONUT PECAN LOAF

Makes 1 loaf

coconut oil, for greasing

2 small or 1 medium sweet potato, peeled and chopped into small pieces

120g buckwheat flour

50g coconut palm sugar, plus extra to sprinkle on top

30g chopped pecan nuts, plus 8–10 whole pecans to garnish

3 tbsp coconut flour

1 1/2 tbsp ground chia seeds

2 tsp ground cinnamon

1/2 tsp baking powder

1 ripe banana

60ml low-fat coconut milk

60ml warm water

1 tsp vanilla extract

This healthy loaf has the sweetness and density of cake thanks to ingredients like cinnamon and sweet potato purée. I love to pair it with smooth almond butter and my raspberry chia jam on page 80 for an easy and delicious breakfast or post-workout snack.

1   Preheat the oven to 190°C. Lightly grease a loaf tin with coconut oil or line the tin with greaseproof paper.
2   Steam the chopped sweet potatoes until soft.
3   Meanwhile, place the buckwheat flour, coconut palm sugar, chopped pecans, coconut flour, chia seeds, cinnamon and baking powder in a large mixing bowl and combine well.
4   Add the steamed sweet potato to a blender with the banana, coconut milk, warm water and vanilla extract and combine until smooth. Add to the dry ingredients and mix well until a dough forms.
5   Place the dough into the prepared loaf tin. Garnish with the whole pecans and a sprinkle of coconut palm sugar.
6   Bake for 25–30 minutes, until golden brown and firm to the touch. Turn out of the tin and allow to cool for 10 minutes on a wire rack. Store in an airtight container in the fridge for up to three days.

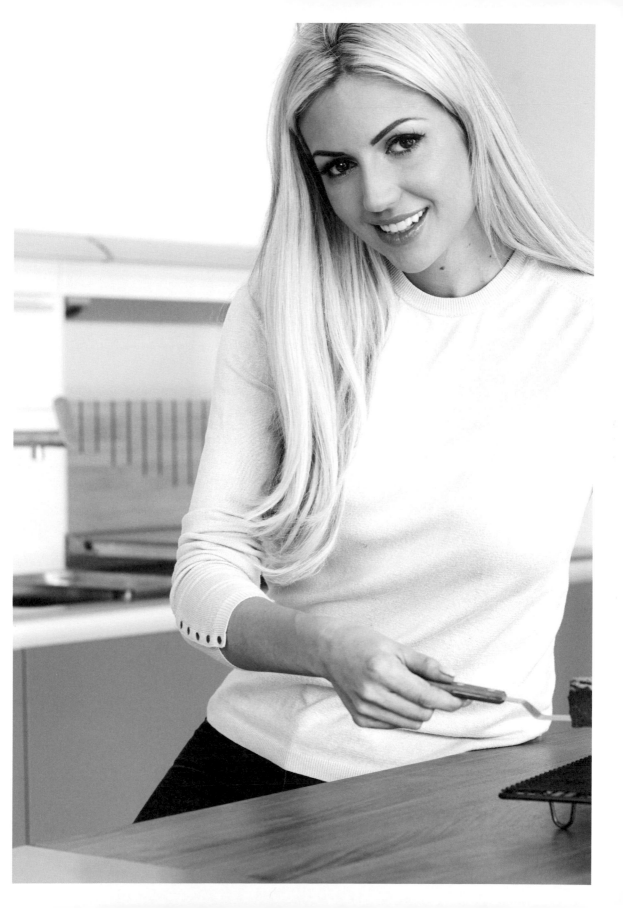

SALADS, SOUPS AND WRAPS

Vibrant vegetables, hearty soups and raw salads will benefit
your skin, health, energy and weight loss more than any other
type of food, so you must focus on this group the most to reach
your highest health and beauty potential. They're bursting
with vitamins, minerals, living enzymes and antioxidants to
reverse the effects of ageing and fill every cell in your body with
nourishment. This group of foods must form the core of the *Eat
Yourself Beautiful* way of life.

Beauty tip:

TRY TO EAT FRESH, RAW OR LIGHTLY **STEAMED GREENS** WITH EACH MEAL FOR THE VERY BEST BEAUTY AND HEALTH RESULTS. I DO THIS BY DRINKING A GREEN GODDESS SMOOTHIE (PAGE 218) IN THE MORNING, MAKING A BIG GREEN SALAD FOR LUNCH AND INCLUDING GREENS LIKE KALE, BROCCOLI OR ASPARAGUS WITH MY EVENING MEAL.

DIGESTION-BOOSTING BASIC GARDEN SALAD

Serves 1

120g leafy greens – I usually opt for a combination of rocket, romaine and butterhead lettuce, but any greens will do

2 tbsp raw apple cider vinegar

juice of $\frac{1}{2}$ lemon

Himalayan pink rock salt and freshly ground black pepper

As the name suggests, the purpose of this salad is to stimulate your digestive juices to properly process any denatured cooked food that you may be eating. I'm a big fan of raw foods and my body often craves them no matter the season. But it's nice to have something hot and comforting on colder nights, so I like to vary my meals. As you know, optimal digestion, including an efficient liver, is the key to the glowing skin and glossy hair. If you're eating cooked meals regularly, then try to get into the habit of eating a simple oil-free green salad as a starter, or piling salad onto your plate to eat before you have the cooked portion. It also helps to fill you up and makes you less likely to overeat. This is one of my top tried-and-tested nutrition tricks for healthy and sustainable fat loss.

1   Wash the greens well in a salad spinner or gently pat dry with kitchen paper. Place in a large bowl and toss with the apple cider vinegar, lemon juice and a pinch of salt and pepper.
2   Transfer to a serving bowl or your dinner plate and enjoy.

MARINATED KALE, AVOCADO AND CITRUS SALAD WITH ROSIE'S CLASSIC DRESSING

Serves 2

270g raw kale (I usually use curly kale)

1 ripe avocado

juice of 1 lemon

Himalayan pink rock salt and freshly ground back pepper

Rosie's classic dressing (page 140), to serve

175g fresh ripe tomatoes, chopped

1 heaped tbsp nutritional yeast

1 tsp chilli flakes (optional)

It may not have a very glamorous name, but this salad will do more for stimulating growth of thick, shiny hair than any expensive product out there. This is also my favourite meal to throw together three or four evenings a week because it's so delicious, filling, quick and nourishing. The kale, avocado and nutritional yeast and the hemp seeds in the dressing contain all of the nutrients needed for luscious locks. Eat this salad regularly and watch your hair grow!

1   Wash the kale well. Remove the tough stems and rip the leaves into smaller pieces. Transfer to a large mixing bowl.
2   Cut the avocado in half lengthways and remove the stone. Scoop out the avocado flesh and add it to the kale along with the lemon juice and seasoning.
3   Now for the fun part! Roll up your sleeves and begin to massage the avocado and lemon juice into the kale. Once the kale is well coated, leave it to marinate for 5–10 minutes while you make the salad dressing on page 140.
4   Transfer the kale to two serving bowls and drizzle the dressing on top. Scatter over the tomatoes, nutritional yeast and chilli flakes and serve.

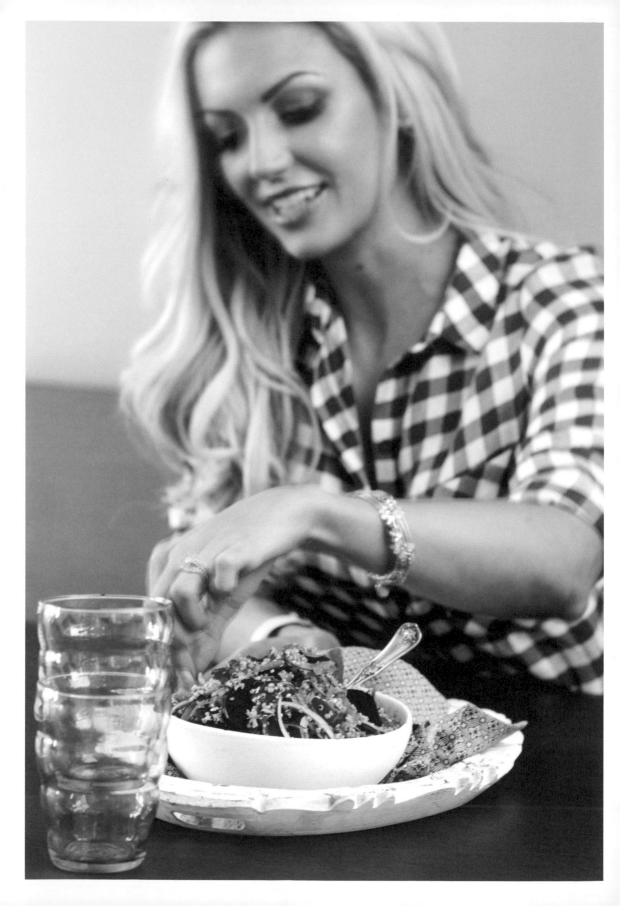

QUINOA AND HEMP SEED COLOUR BOWL

Serves 2

170g quinoa

500ml low-sodium vegetable stock

80g black or green olives, stoned

2 large, ripe tomatoes, chopped

2 medium carrots, peeled and grated

1 cooked beetroot, finely sliced

$\frac{1}{2}$ red onion, finely sliced

2 cloves of garlic, minced

3 tbsp chopped fresh coriander

2 tbsp sunflower seeds

2 tbsp hulled hemp seeds

2 tsp smoked paprika

1 tsp finely grated fresh ginger

juice of 1 lime

Himalayan pink rock salt and freshly ground black pepper

1 tbsp chopped fresh mint

This simple, nutrient-rich quinoa and mixed veggie dish is a firm favourite of mine as it serves as another little reminder to eat your daily quota of colourful vegetables. Packed with complete plant protein, fibre, omega-3 and omega-6 fats, vitamins and minerals, it's easy to whip up in under half an hour. Promise!

1   Rinse the quinoa well in a sieve. Put the vegetable stock into a medium saucepan. Bring it to the boil and add in the quinoa. Stir well, cover and lower the heat. Allow it to simmer for 15–20 minutes, until the quinoa seeds have opened out. Remove the quinoa from the heat and keep it covered to soak up any remaining stock for 5–10 minutes.

2   Prepare the vegetables while the quinoa is cooking.

3   Place the cooked quinoa in a large bowl and fluff it up with a fork before adding the olives, tomatoes, carrots, beetroot, onion, garlic, coriander, sunflower seeds, hemp seeds, smoked paprika and ginger. Mix together well. Drizzle with lime juice and add seasoning to taste.

4   Transfer to two serving bowls, scatter over the fresh mint and serve straightaway.

HAPPY SKIN
TABBOULEH SALAD

Serves 3–4

60g fresh flat-leaf parsley

4 tbsp fresh mint leaves

1 clove of garlic, peeled

pinch of Himalayan pink
rock salt

150g hulled hemp seeds

150g cherry tomatoes, halved

juice of 2 limes (about 2 tbsp)

1 tsp smoked paprika

freshly ground black pepper

$^1/_2$ tsp dried chilli flakes

Rich in essential amino acids, beauty vitamins and minerals, healthy fats, detoxifying parsley and lime juice, this simple but powerful salad is up there with my favourite dishes of all time! While traditional Lebanese tabbouleh is made with bulgur wheat, I have used hulled hemp seeds for their incredible smoothing benefits to your skin due to their impressive essential omega-3 fat content.

1   Whizz the parsley, mint, garlic and a pinch of salt in a blender or food processor until well combined.
2   Pour into a mixing bowl, then add the hemp seeds, cherry tomatoes, lime juice, smoked paprika and some freshly ground black pepper and stir well.
3   Transfer to serving bowls, top with the chilli flakes and serve.

ANTI-AGEING MAURITIAN SALAD

Serves 2

200g mixed salad leaves

150g fresh pineapple chunks

150g cherry tomatoes, halved

60g walnut halves

30g unsweetened
coconut flakes

1 large, ripe avocado, pitted,
peeled and sliced

4 tbsp freshly squeezed
lemon juice

2 tbsp low-sodium tamari

2 tbsp chopped fresh
mint leaves

freshly ground black pepper

pinch of dried chilli flakes
(optional)

I have been visiting Mauritius annually with my family for the past 20 years, and if there's one thing we've noticed, it's that the people there don't seem to age a day! No doubt the more relaxed pace of life helps, but their diets seem to be rich in wholesome raw fruit and veggies, which really are key to holding back the years. This salad is inspired by my favourite lunch served at the hotel we stay in, and I order it almost every single day of the holiday. It's such a great combination of tropical flavours, anti-inflammatory pineapple and greens, and skin-smoothing healthy fats from the avocado, walnuts and coconut.

1   Wash the greens well and dry in a salad spinner or gently pat dry with kitchen paper.
2   Place the greens in a large mixing bowl with the pineapple, cherry tomatoes, walnuts, coconut flakes and avocado. Drizzle over the lemon juice and tamari and toss to combine.
3   Divide the salad between two plates or bowls. Top with the mint leaves, some freshly ground black pepper and a pinch of chilli flakes, if using.

RAINBOW GLOW BOWL

Serves 2

150g cherry tomatoes, halved

2 carrots sliced into sticks

2 radishes, thinly sliced

1 yellow or red pepper, deseeded and sliced

1 ripe avocado, pitted, peeled and sliced

4 tbsp purple power slaw salad (page 122)

2 tbsp vegan basil pesto (page 149)

2 tbsp raw pumpkin seeds, to garnish

2 tsp smoked paprika, to garnish

pinch of dried chilli flakes, to garnish

FOR THE TURMERIC QUINOA:

170g quinoa

500ml water

1 heaped tsp ground turmeric

Himalayan pink rock salt and freshly ground black pepper

We're always told to eat a rainbow of colourful raw fruits and vegetables each day to benefit from their wide range of healing antioxidants. For younger-looking skin that's glowing with good health, I whip together a rainbow glow bowl at least once a week for a nourishing lunch. It can be whatever selection of different dips and veggies you fancy, but my favourites include purple power slaw salad (page 122), cherry tomatoes, avocado, chopped carrot, yellow and red peppers, turmeric quinoa,* pumpkin seeds and a dollop of vegan basil pesto (page 149).

1 To prepare the turmeric quinoa, first rinse the quinoa well in a sieve. Bring the water to a low boil in a saucepan set over a medium heat. Add the quinoa and allow it to boil for 2 minutes before taking the temperature down, partly covering the saucepan with a lid and leaving it to simmer for 10–15 minutes, until the quinoa seeds have opened.

2 Remove from the heat and stir in the turmeric and some salt and pepper. Cover the saucepan and allow it to sit for another 10 minutes to absorb any remaining liquid. When it's ready, fluff up the quinoa with a fork.

3 Assemble the raw vegetables around the edges of a large plate or shallow bowl. Place a serving of the turmeric quinoa, the purple power slaw salad and a dollop of the vegan basil pesto in the middle.

4 Garnish with the pumpkin seeds, smoked paprika and dried chilli flakes and serve.

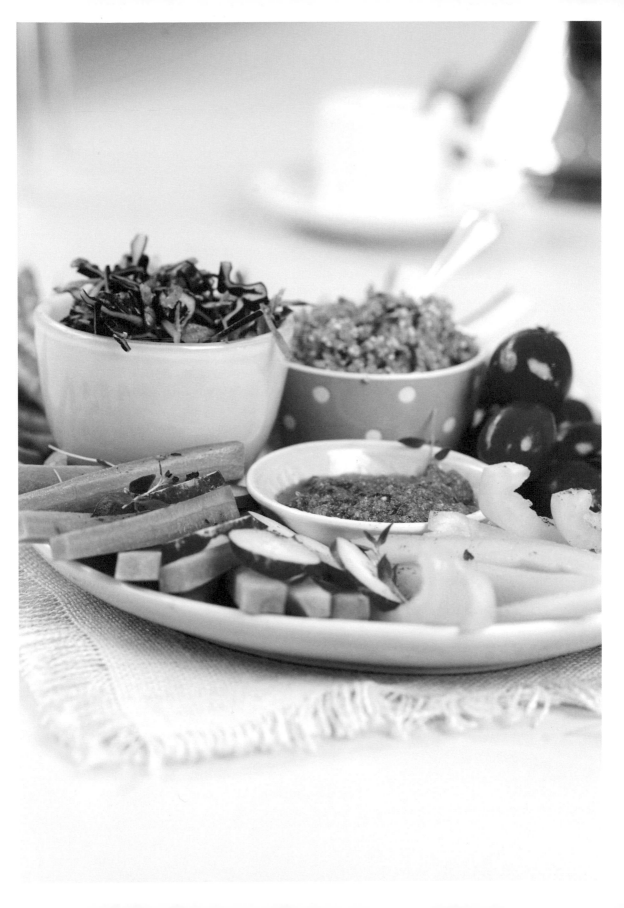

BRIGHT-EYED CHICKPEA AND CARROT SALAD WITH GINGER SESAME DRESSING

Serves 3–4

1 courgette

4 large carrots

250g cooked chickpeas (see page 22 for cooking instructions)

120g fresh parsley, long stems removed and leaves chopped

40g pumpkin seeds

ginger sesame dressing (page 141)

Himalayan pink rock salt and freshly ground black pepper

1 tsp lemon zest, to garnish

Did your mother ever tell you to eat up all your carrots to help you see in the dark? I definitely heard that line across the dinner table on more than one occasion. While it isn't entirely true, carrots do contain plenty of beta-carotene, which your body converts to vitamin A. This vitamin then helps your eyes to convert light so that it can be transmitted to your brain, enabling you to see better in low light. In extreme cases, a vitamin A deficiency can lead to blindness, so it's always a good idea to include brightly coloured fruit and veggies like carrots in your diet as frequently as you can.

1   Wash the courgette and top and tail it. I like to use a spiral-iser to grate it and the carrots into ribbons, but a vegetable peeler also works.
2   Place the courgette and carrot ribbons, chickpeas, parsley and pumpkin seeds in a large mixing bowl.
3   Drizzle the ginger sesame dressing over the salad, add some seasoning to taste and toss together well.
4   Garnish with the fresh lemon zest and serve.

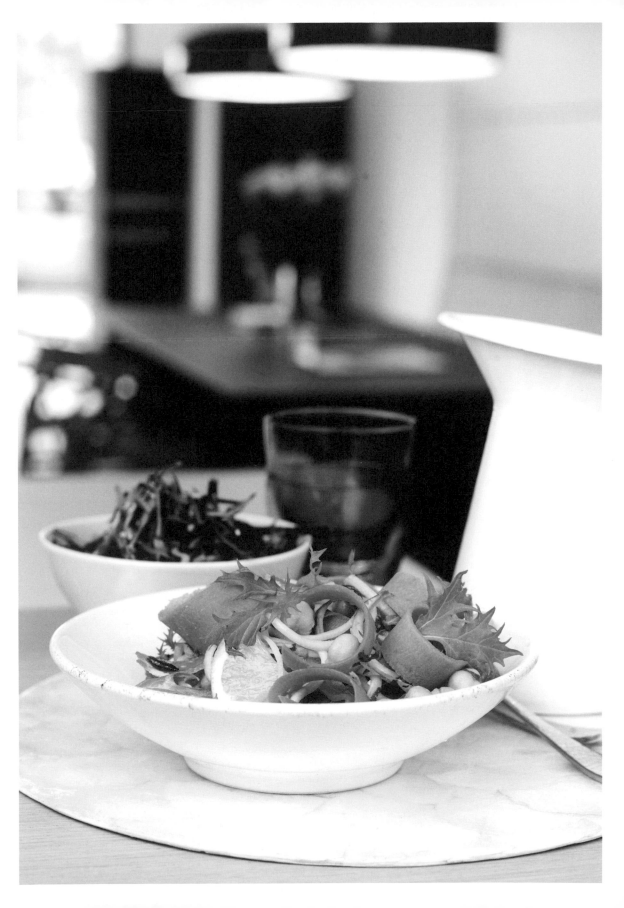

VEGAN CAESAR SALAD

Serves 2–3

1 bag of kale (I use curly kale)

12 cherry tomatoes, halved

3 heaped tbsp nutritional yeast

FOR THE CHICKPEA 'CROUTONS':

250g cooked chickpeas (see page 22 for cooking instructions)

2 tbsp organic virgin coconut oil, melted

1 tsp smoked paprika

pinch of cayenne pepper

FOR THE DRESSING:

40g raw cashew nuts

1 clove of garlic, peeled

juice of 1 lemon

2 tbsp hulled hemp seeds

2 tsp cold-pressed extra virgin olive oil

Himalayan pink rock salt and freshly ground black pepper

My husband loves a good Caesar salad because it's hearty enough to fill him up and keep him going for the afternoon. However, traditional Caesar salads contain less healthy ingredients like cheese and oily croutons, which can be a digestive disaster. This recipe still offers all the satisfying creaminess of a Caesar salad, but I've added ingredients like chickpea 'croutons', hemp seeds and nutritional yeast, which give it plenty of flavour but help to balance out blood sugar levels and boost your omega-3 fats. I also use kale to top up your daily dose of fibre to keep you feeling energised all afternoon long, plus calcium, iron and other essential beauty nutrients.

1 To make the dressing, soak the cashews in a bowl of cold water for 2–3 hours. Drain well.

2 Put the soaked cashews, garlic, lemon juice, hemp seeds, olive oil and some salt and pepper in a blender or food processor. Slowly add in some water as you blend with the motor running until you've achieved your preferred consistency. Pour the dressing into a container and store in the fridge while you put together the rest of the salad.

3 To make the chickpea 'croutons', preheat the oven to 200°C.

4 Place the chickpeas on a baking tray, drizzle with the melted coconut oil and sprinkle with the smoked paprika, a pinch of cayenne and some salt and pepper. Ensure all the chickpeas are coated well in the oil and spices.

5 Bake the chickpeas in the oven for 25–30 minutes, until they turn golden brown and crisp. Stir them every 10–15 minutes to ensure they don't burn. Set aside to cool.

6 To prepare the salad, wash the kale well and remove the thick stems. Pat the leaves dry with kitchen paper or in a salad spinner, then tear the leaves into smaller pieces.

7 Place the kale in a large mixing bowl and pour over your desired quantity of Caesar dressing. To soften the kale, I like to use my hands to massage the dressing into the leaves. Leave for 5 minutes to allow the kale to soak up the dressing.

8 Add the cherry tomatoes and chickpea 'croutons'. Sprinkle with the nutritional yeast and serve.

RAW PROBIOTIC SEED AND FENNEL CHEESE

Serves 3–4

150g sunflower seeds

120g pumpkin seeds

1/2 medium red onion, finely sliced

1 tbsp fennel seeds

2 capsules of Udo's Choice Super 8 probiotics, split to release the powder inside

Himalayan pink rock salt and freshly ground black pepper

This mixed seed cheese is a good alternative for all the milk-based cheese addicts out there. I should know, because I used to be one! It was the thought of giving up cheese that actually prevented me from going from vegetarian to vegan for a long time because, like many people I know and work with, I didn't think I could cope without it in my life. But of course I felt so much better when I gave it up that I didn't need any more convincing. My problem skin cleared up, my digestion improved and pounds melted off my frame even though I was eating more (plant-based) food than ever before. In this dairy-free cheese I've added all-important probiotics in the form of powder from capsules and I've added flavour with onion and fennel seeds. Fennel is a powerful antioxidant and anti-inflammatory spice. I eat the cheese on salads and in soups and I use it as a dip for raw veggie sticks.

1   Place the sunflower and pumpkin seeds in a large bowl or jar and fill with water to completely submerge them. Cover and leave to soak overnight.

2   The next day, drain the liquid and rinse the seeds in fresh water.

3   Using a blender, combine the soaked seeds with the onion, fennel seeds, probiotics and some salt and pepper until it's almost smooth. Use a little water to help it blend if necessary.

4   Pour the mixture into a large glass jar or jug, cover with a cheesecloth and let it sit at room temperature for 4–5 hours to allow the probiotics to start fermenting the cheese. It will rise slightly as it ferments.

5   If you prefer a softer, ricotta-like texture, then simply leave the cheese as it is in the jar. But if you would rather have a firmer cheese, then after it has been fermenting for 2 hours, secure the cheesecloth with an elastic band and turn the entire jar or jug upside down over a bowl to strain out any remaining liquid. Leave it in this position for the final 2–3 hours.

6   Remove the cheese from the container, wrap in greaseproof paper and keep refrigerated for up to one week.

BAKED ITALIAN HERB CHEESE

Serves 4

220g raw unsalted almonds

2 cloves of garlic, chopped

120ml water, to blend

60ml freshly squeezed lemon juice

3 tbsp extra virgin olive oil

1 tsp dried Italian herbs

$1/_2$ tsp unpasteurised miso paste

pinch of cayenne pepper

pinch of Himalayan pink rock salt

coconut oil, for greasing

This delicately flavoured almond cheese works well as a cheese substitute and you can add whatever herbs and spices you please. It's delicious on salads and with my wheat-free bread (page 95). Cheese addicts, rejoice!

1 Soak the almonds in a bowl of cold water for 6–8 hours or overnight. Make sure the almonds are covered with at least 2.5cm of water so that they stay covered with water as they swell.

2 Drain and rinse the almonds in fresh water. Place them in a blender or food processor with the rest of the ingredients (except the coconut oil) and blend until smooth.

3 Pour the cheese mixture into a cheesecloth or piece of muslin and place it in a strainer or sieve set over a bowl. Leave in the fridge overnight. Save the liquid that drains off, as it works well as a salad dressing!

4 The next day, preheat the oven to 180°C. Lightly grease a 20cm x 12cm loaf tin with coconut oil.

5 Place the drained cheese mixture in the greased tin. Bake the cheese in the oven for 40–45 minutes, until it's firm to touch and the top is beginning to turn golden brown and crisp. Remove from the oven and allow to cool for 10 minutes.

6 Serve warm or cold with salads, my wheat-free bread (page 95) or crackers. Store in the fridge for up to three days in an airtight container.

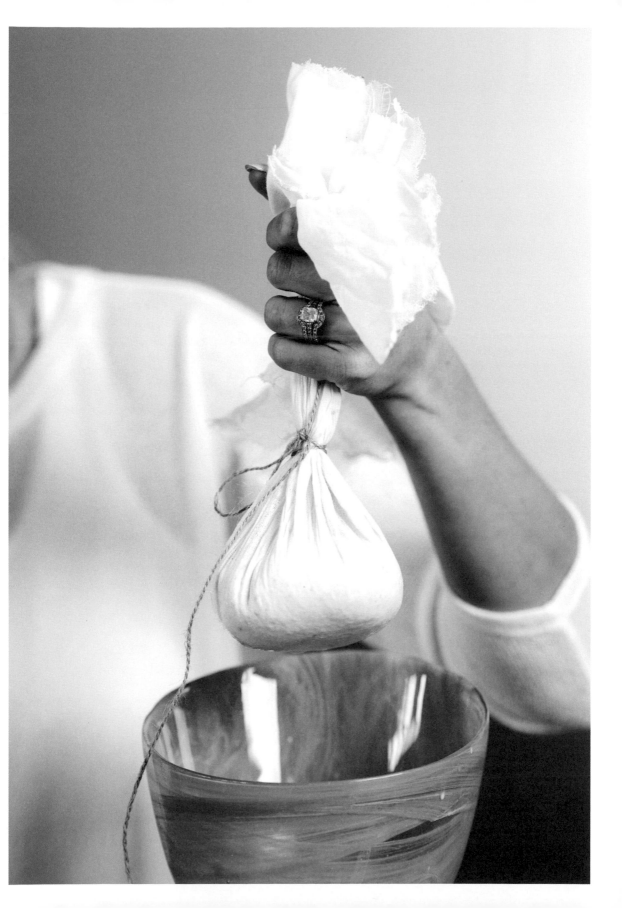

COLLAGEN-BUILDING PURPLE POWER SLAW WITH CITRUS TAHINI DRESSING

Serves 2

400g red cabbage (about ¹/₂ medium head), finely shredded

2 carrots, peeled and grated

1 large or 2 small cooked beetroots, grated or finely sliced

1 red onion, finely sliced

1 large orange, peeled and segmented

Himalayan pink rock salt and freshly ground black pepper

2 heaped tbsp sesame seeds, toasted

citrus tahini dressing (page 141)

Eaten regularly, this simple salad can have a powerful impact on your appearance, especially the collagen in your skin, thanks to the high levels of vitamin C in the cabbage and orange. The beta-carotene in the carrots also helps to build a radiant complexion, while the beetroot is known for its deep-cleansing and blood-building properties. I love this bright orange and purple salad with the creaminess of my citrus tahini dressing, which also aids in the absorption of its fat-soluble vitamins.

1   Place the cabbage in a large mixing bowl with the grated carrots, beetroot and onion.
2   Cut each orange segment in half and add to the vegetables. Add some seasoning to taste and mix well.
3   Toast the sesame seeds in a small, dry pan over a medium heat just until they start to turn golden. Take care not to burn them.
4   Drizzle with citrus tahini dressing, sprinkle with the toasted sesame seeds and serve.

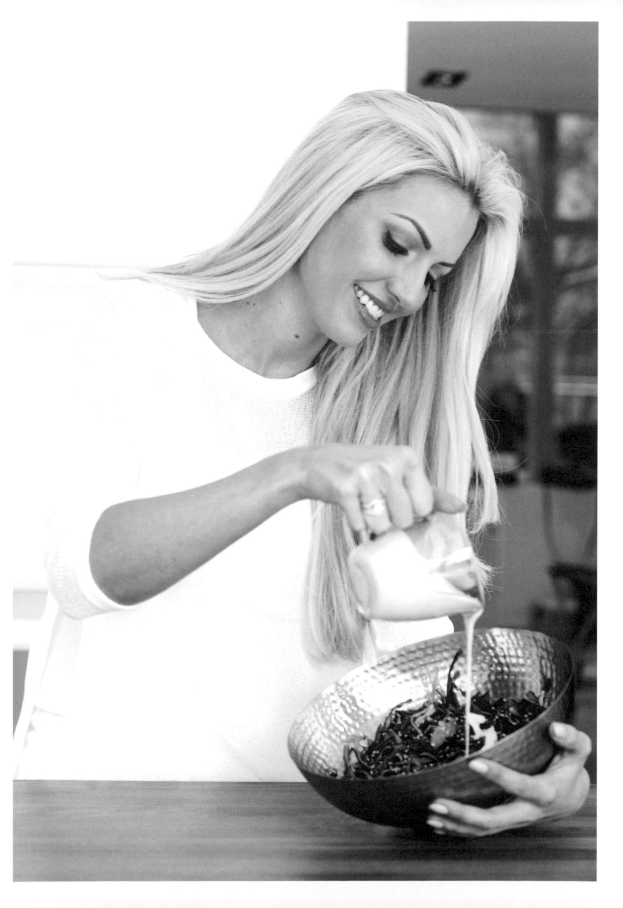

TUMMY-FLATTENING GINGER AND CARAWAY SAUERKRAUT

Serves 2

1 medium head of red cabbage

950ml water

2 tbsp peeled and chopped fresh ginger

1 tbsp unpasteurised miso paste

1 heaped tbsp caraway seeds

A centuries-long tradition in many cultures, fermented foods and drinks, such as sauerkraut, kimchi and coconut water kefir, are one of the ultimate secrets to a lifetime of glowing beauty and health. Seriously! The most significant change I have ever seen in my own health, skin and body was when I started including probiotic-rich sauerkraut and kefir in my diet on a regular basis. The friendly bacteria in fermented foods really help to improve digestion for a flatter stomach, and nutrient absorption greatly improves for healthier skin and hair. Improved mental clarity, calmness and a much stronger immune system are added benefits. It makes sense considering that 80% of our immune system and 90% of our serotonin production are based in our gut. Though I do take probiotic capsules when I'm travelling, when I'm at home I drink my own home-brewed kefir and make a batch of sauerkraut once or twice a week. Made from the humble cabbage, raw sauerkraut is a great option for beginners, as kefir requires a starter pack of 'grains'. I love how simple this recipe is – most of the work is done when the cabbage is left to gently ferment and generate beneficial bacteria. I pile it on top of nori wraps and salads and eat it as a side dish with curries and quinoa dishes, as the ginger and caraway flavours lend themselves well to other spiced dishes.

1   You'll need two or three 1–1.5 litre glass mason or Kilner
    jars with airtight lids to ferment the cabbage over four to
    five days, and they must be well sealed. The jars and lids
    also must be spotlessly clean and sterilised. If you have a
    dishwasher, you can simply run everything through a hot
    cycle. Otherwise, wash everything in hot, soapy water, rinse
    well, then place the jars and lids on a baking tray in an oven
    heated to 140°C and keep them there until you're ready to
    use them.

2   Remove the tough outer leaves from the cabbage and set
    them to one side to use later. Shred the cabbage in a food
    processor or with a sharp knife until it's finely sliced.

3   Combine the water, ginger and miso paste in a blender and
    whizz until smooth. Add the caraway seeds once it's blended.

4   Evenly distribute the cabbage between the sterilised jars
    and pour over the miso liquid. Using a large spoon, press
    down firmly on the cabbage to ensure it's tightly packed
    into the jars. Leave 5cm of space clear at the top of each jar.
    Place one of the tough outer leaves of cabbage on top of
    each jar to fill the 5cm of space. Screw the lids onto the jars
    tightly.

5   To ferment the cabbage, leave the jars in a warm, dark place
    for five days. The ideal temperature is 19–24°C. You may
    notice some bubbles in the jars, and that's a good sign that
    the cabbage is fermenting. After five days, move the jars to
    the fridge to slow down the fermentation process.

6   When ready to serve, simply remove the tough cabbage leaf
    from the top of the jar and scoop out the sauerkraut.

7   Keep the jars stored in the fridge. The sauerkraut will stay
    fresh for up to four weeks after you open the jar and can be
    kept unopened for up to three months in the fridge.

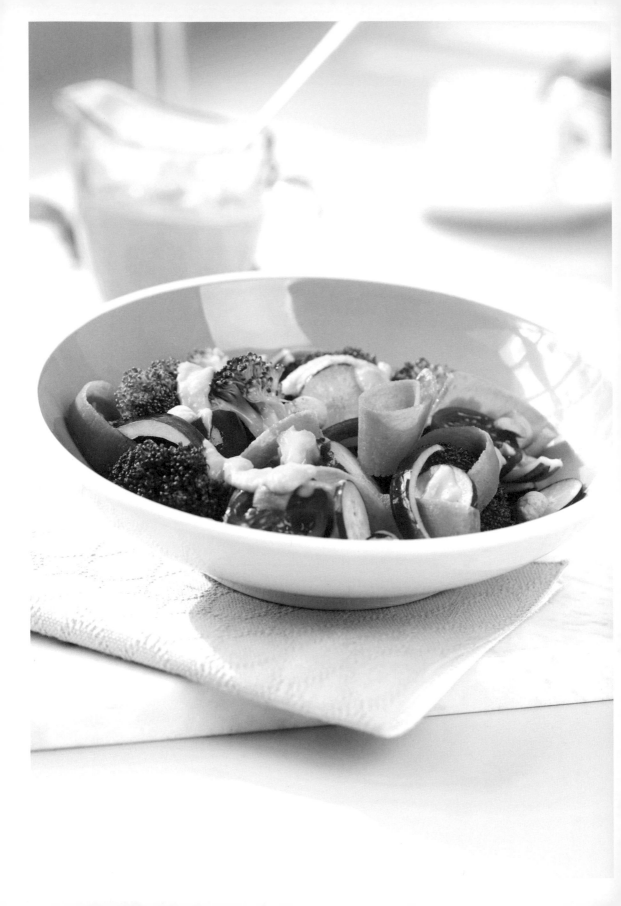

PHYTONUTRIENT GLOW SALAD WITH CREAMY AVOCADO DRESSING

Serves 2

175g skinned hazelnuts, halved

1 head of broccoli, cut into small bite-sized florets

150g cherry tomatoes, halved

2 radishes, thinly sliced

2 carrots, peeled into ribbons

1 medium red onion, finely sliced

juice of 1 lime

pinch of dried chilli flakes (optional)

Himalayan pink rock salt and freshly ground black pepper

2 tbsp chopped fresh mint leaves

creamy avocado dressing (page 142)

In terms of fighting disease and filling you up with protective phytonutrients, vitamins and minerals like vitamins C, K and A, calcium and iron, broccoli is one of the most impressive vegetables there is for maintaining our beauty and health. But I had never been a big fan of eating raw broccoli until I created this recipe. The tangy lime, the fresh mint and the creaminess of the avocado dressing really lift the broccoli, making it a refreshing, light, crunchy salad. I've added some sliced raw radishes because they contain the magical trio of silica, sulphur and vitamin C, which work in synergy for glowing skin.

1 Preheat the oven to 190°C.
2 Spread out the hazelnuts on a baking tray and place in the oven for 5–10 minutes, until lightly toasted. Set side to cool.
3 Place the broccoli florets in a salad serving bowl with the halved cherry tomatoes, sliced radishes, carrot ribbons and sliced red onion. Drizzle the lime juice on top, sprinkle with a pinch of chilli flakes (if using) and season to taste with salt and pepper. Toss together well.
4 Drizzle the creamy avocado dressing on top. Sprinkle with the fresh chopped mint and toasted hazelnuts and serve.

LONG LOCKS LENTIL AND ROAST MUSHROOM SALAD

Serves 2

FOR THE LENTIL SALAD:

200g Puy lentils

1 tbsp organic virgin coconut oil

1 red onion, diced

1/2 red pepper, diced

2 cloves of garlic, minced

Himalayan pink rock salt and freshly ground black pepper

75g organic baby spinach, washed

2 tbsp freshly squeezed lemon juice

2 tbsp chopped fresh coriander, to garnish

pinch of dried chilli flakes, to garnish

FOR THE MARINATED MUSHROOMS:

4 Portobello mushrooms, rinsed well

1/4 red onion, diced

60ml balsamic vinegar

2 tbsp minced fresh garlic

1 tbsp organic virgin coconut oil, melted, plus extra for greasing

1 tbsp freshly squeezed lemon juice

1 tsp dried thyme

1 tsp dried basil

pinch of dried chilli flakes

Himalayan pink rock salt and freshly ground black pepper

Packed with easily assimilated plant protein, minerals such as iron and zinc plus plenty of B vitamins and folate, this is another great dish for optimising your hair growth and health.

1   Place the mushrooms in a sealable plastic sandwich bag or ziplock bag. Combine all the marinade ingredients in a small bowl and mix together well. Pour the marinade into the bag with the mushrooms, seal well and shake it gently to coat the mushrooms in the marinade. Lie the bag flat and marinate the mushrooms for 1–5 hours at room temperature, shaking the bag occasionally to keep the mushrooms evenly coated.

2   Preheat the oven to 200°C. Lightly grease a baking tray with coconut oil.

3   Remove the mushrooms from the marinade and place on the greased baking tray. Roast for 20–25 minutes, turning them over after 10 minutes.

4   While the mushrooms are roasting, prepare the lentil salad. To cook the lentils, first rinse them in a sieve under cold running water. Transfer them to a medium saucepan and cover with double their volume of water. Over a medium-high heat, bring the lentils to a rapid simmer and then reduce the temperature to gently simmer them, uncovered, for 20–30 minutes. The lentils should be just barely covered with water and are cooked once they're tender rather than crunchy.

5   Heat the coconut oil in a saucepan over a medium heat. Lightly sauté the onion, red pepper and garlic for 5 minutes, until they begin to soften. Add the cooked lentils and gently heat them through. Add seasoning to taste.

6   Place a bed of baby spinach on a serving plate and arrange the lentils on top.

7   With a sharp knife, cut the roasted mushrooms into strips and scatter them across the lentil salad. Add a little more seasoning and the fresh lemon juice. Garnish with the fresh coriander and dried chilli flakes and serve warm.

COCONUT AND QUINOA CURRIED LENTIL SOUP

Serves 3–4

1 tbsp organic coconut oil

1 large onion, diced

2 cloves of garlic, finely chopped

1 tbsp finely chopped fresh ginger

2 tbsp curry powder

2 tbsp tomato paste

$\frac{1}{2}$ tsp chilli flakes

180g ripe tomatoes, diced

130g red lentils

1 litre low-sodium vegetable stock

250ml low-fat coconut milk

Himalayan pink rock salt and freshly ground black pepper

85g quinoa

250ml water

60g fresh baby spinach

2 tbsp chopped fresh coriander, to garnish

This soup is a warming lunch, dinner or snack. Lentils are extremely affordable and are the perfect source of plant-based protein, fibre and antioxidants. They also keep you feeling full for hours and are more digestible than other types of legumes. Quinoa is a gluten-free source of high-quality plant protein without the cholesterol and saturated fat. It contains all eight essential amino acids plus plenty of magnesium, fibre, manganese, calcium and phosphorus as well as B vitamins and iron to boost energy.

1   Heat the coconut oil in a saucepan over a medium heat. Sauté the onion, garlic and ginger for a couple of minutes. Add the curry powder, tomato paste and chilli flakes and cook for another 1–2 minutes. Add the diced tomatoes, lentils, vegetable stock and coconut milk. Cover and bring to the boil, then reduce the heat to low and simmer for 20–30 minutes, until the lentils are tender. Season with salt and pepper to taste.

2   Rinse the quinoa well in a sieve and place it in a separate medium saucepan. Add the water, cover the pan and set over a medium heat. Bring the quinoa to a boil for 5 minutes, then cover the pan, reduce the heat and simmer for 10–15 minutes, until the seeds have opened out. Remove the lid and stir the quinoa with a fork until the rest of the water has evaporated.

3   Remove the lentil soup from the heat. Stir in the spinach and allow it to wilt. Add the quinoa to the soup and stir well.

4   Ladle into soup bowls and garnish with the chopped coriander. Serve hot.

IMMUNITY-BOOSTING BUTTERNUT SQUASH, GINGER AND COCONUT SOUP

Serves 2

1 butternut squash, washed and left whole

1 tbsp organic virgin coconut oil, plus extra for greasing

1 red pepper

1/2 red onion, chopped

2 cloves of garlic, minced

1 tbsp finely chopped fresh ginger

700ml low-sodium vegetable stock

150ml low-fat coconut milk

2 tsp smoked paprika

1 tsp ground turmeric

1 tsp dried chilli flakes

Himalayan pink rock salt and freshly ground black pepper

2 tbsp chopped fresh coriander, to garnish

2 tbsp pumpkin seeds, to garnish

Butternut squash is such a versatile, filling and inexpensive vegetable, full of health- and beauty-enhancing fibre, vitamins, minerals and antioxidants. This soup is one of my favourite ways to eat the root vegetable and it's so easy to make – all you need is a blender. I love adding the turmeric, ginger and a pinch of chilli flakes for a warming and immune-boosting meal.

1   Preheat the oven to 200°C. Lightly grease a baking tray with coconut oil.

2   Place the whole squash on the greased baking tray. Bake for 20–25 minutes, until it has started to soften and the skin is turning golden brown. Remove from the oven, and when it's cool enough to handle, cut it open and remove the seeds. Peel off the skin and cut the squash into chunks.

3   Heat the coconut oil in a saucepan over a medium heat. Sauté the red pepper, onion, garlic and ginger for about 5 minutes, until the onion is lightly browned.

4   Place the chopped butternut squash, sautéed vegetables, vegetable stock, coconut milk, smoked paprika, turmeric, chilli flakes and some salt and pepper into a blender or use a hand-held stick blender. Blend until smooth.

5   Ladle into soup bowls and garnish with the chopped coriander and a sprinkle of pumpkin seeds. Serve hot.

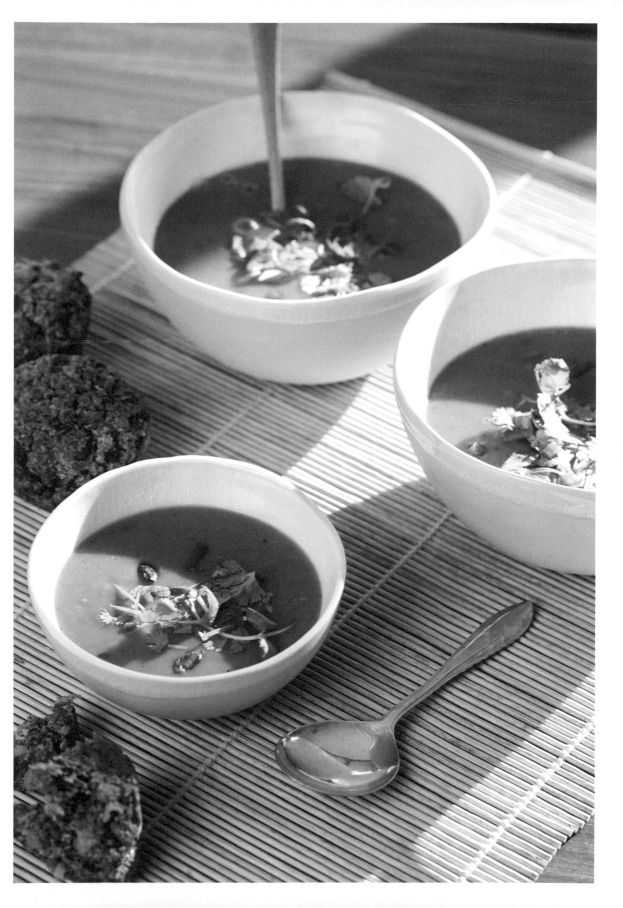

WARMING APPLE AND VEGETABLE SOUP

Serves 2–3

1 tbsp coconut oil

1 large onion, diced

2 cloves of garlic, roughly chopped

2 small fresh red chillies, deseeded and chopped

2 tsp medium curry powder

2 tsp ground turmeric

1 tsp ground cumin

1 tsp ground coriander

pink Himalayan rock salt and freshly ground black pepper

2 carrots, peeled and chopped into chunks

1 courgette, sliced

1 small sweet potato, peeled and chopped

1 medium cooking apple, peeled, cored and chopped

125g runner beans, trimmed

50g red lentils

700ml low-sodium vegetable stock

150ml low-fat coconut milk

2 tbsp apple cider vinegar

This is a recipe that my mum originally made for me one chilly November afternoon when I called by for lunch. I loved the combination of earthy root veggies and tangy apple, so I asked her for the recipe and adapted it slightly to give it a curry twist. I also added the anti-inflammatory spice turmeric, which helps to brighten your skin and give you a healthy glow when eaten regularly. Low in fat and high in fibre and nourishment, this is a great meal or snack option.

1   Heat the coconut oil in a saucepan on a medium heat. Add the onion, garlic, chillies, curry powder, turmeric, cumin, coriander and seasoning and lightly brown for 1–2 minutes, until the spices are fragrant.

2   Add the carrots, courgette, sweet potato, apple, runner beans and lentils and cook for another 3–4 minutes, stirring regularly, until everything starts to soften.

3   Stir in the vegetable stock, coconut milk and apple cider vinegar. Bring the soup to a boil for 5 minutes, then cover the pan, reduce the heat and simmer gently for 15–20 minutes, until the vegetables soften. Transfer the soup to a blender or use a hand-held blender to purée the soup.

4   Serve immediately, or it will keep in the fridge for up to four days and in the freezer for up to six months.

ANTI-ACNE THAI-SPICED PUMPKIN SOUP

Serves 2–3

2 tsp organic virgin coconut oil

1kg pumpkin, peeled and chopped into chunks

1 red onion, finely chopped

4 cloves of garlic, minced or finely chopped

1 tbsp chopped fresh ginger

500ml vegetable stock

500ml low-fat coconut milk

1 tbsp curry powder (add more if you like a curry flavour)

1 tsp smoked paprika, plus extra to garnish

$^1/_2$ tsp dried thyme

$^1/_2$ tsp ground nutmeg

pinch of cayenne pepper (more if you like it spicy)

Himalayan pink rock salt and freshly ground black pepper

2 tbsp chopped fresh parsley, to garnish

1 tbsp pumpkin seeds, to garnish

There are few dishes more ideal than this one for a warming and nourishing lunch or light dinner. Plus it's seriously easy to make, yet looks rather impressive when served in its decoratively carved pumpkin shell placed in the centre of the table. All you need is a few bowls, a ladle and some seedy brown (gluten-free) bread. Pumpkins are low in calories yet packed with fibre to help you feel full for longer. They also have plenty of vitamins and minerals to help you glow from the inside out. They're rich in zinc, which protects your immune system and is crucial for clear, healthy skin and for reducing acne. Pumpkins' high levels of beta-carotene and other antioxidants build youthful skin by protecting your cells against the free radicals that cause premature ageing. Pumpkins can even help you to feel more positive and sleep better too thanks to the amino acid tryptophan, which is a co-factor in producing the 'happy hormone', serotonin, and the sleep hormone, melatonin.

1   Heat the coconut oil in a saucepan on a medium heat. Add the pumpkin, onion, garlic and ginger and cook for 4–5 minutes, stirring frequently so it doesn't burn.

2   Add the stock, coconut milk, spices and seasoning. Partly cover the saucepan with a lid and bring to a boil for 5 minutes, then reduce the heat and simmer for 15–20 minutes, until the pumpkin is soft. Add more stock if necessary.

3   Take off the heat and either pour the soup into a blender or use a hand-held soup blender to whizz it all together until smooth. Taste it at this point to see if it needs any more herbs, spices or seasoning.

4   Pour into soup bowls or a hollowed-out pumpkin shell. Garnish with the chopped parsley, pumpkin seeds and a sprinkle of smoked paprika.

NORI RAINBOW WRAPS WITH GINGER SESAME DRESSING

Serves 2

4 large nori sheets

4 large, soft, flat lettuce leaves (I like to use butterhead lettuce)

4 tbsp lemon and parsley hummus (page 145)

1 ripe avocado, pitted, peeled and sliced

1 carrot, peeled and grated

1 red or yellow bell pepper, deseeded and sliced

4 sugar snap peas, sliced

1/2 medium red onion, finely sliced

4 tbsp chopped fresh coriander

Himalayan pink rock salt and freshly ground black pepper

ginger sesame dressing (page 141)

It's a good idea to regularly include sea veggies in your diet for their beautifying essential minerals and their thyroid- and metabolism-boosting benefits. This is one of my favourite ways to eat nori sheets, featuring a rainbow of colourful veggies, and my protein-packed lemon and parsley hummus and calcium-rich ginger sesame dressing.

1   Lay out each nori sheet on a flat surface. Place a lettuce leaf on top of each sheet to form the wrap.
2   Spread 1 tablespoon of hummus along the side of the wrap closest to you, leaving a gap clear between the hummus and the edge of the wrap.
3   Arrange the avocado, carrot, pepper, peas, onion and 1 table-spoon of chopped coriander in a neat line along the middle of the wrap and season with salt and pepper.
4   Carefully roll up the sheet, beginning with the side nearest you. Seal the nori with a little water. Using a sharp knife, carefully cut the wraps into individual pieces.
5   Arrange the wraps on two serving plates and drizzle with the ginger sesame dressing.

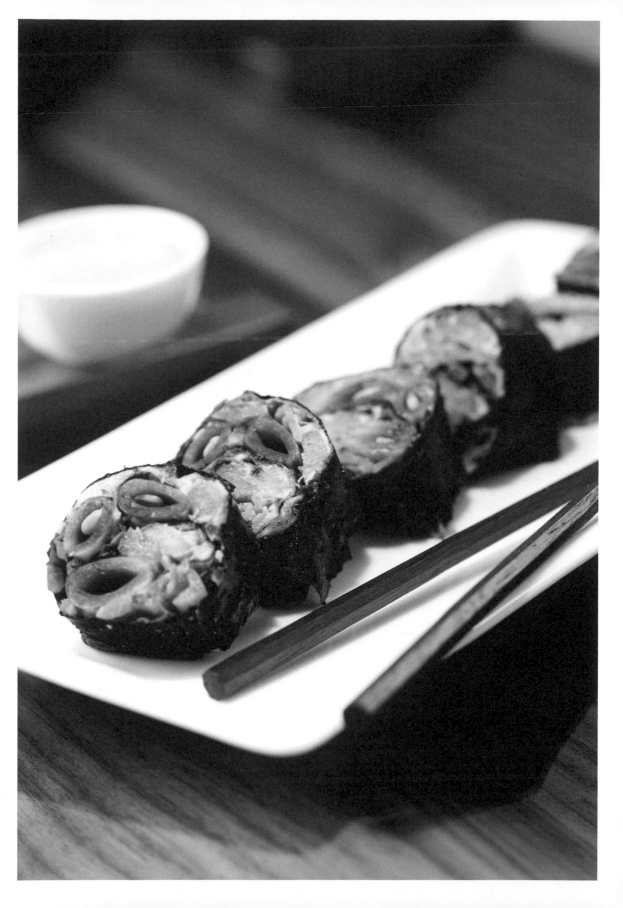

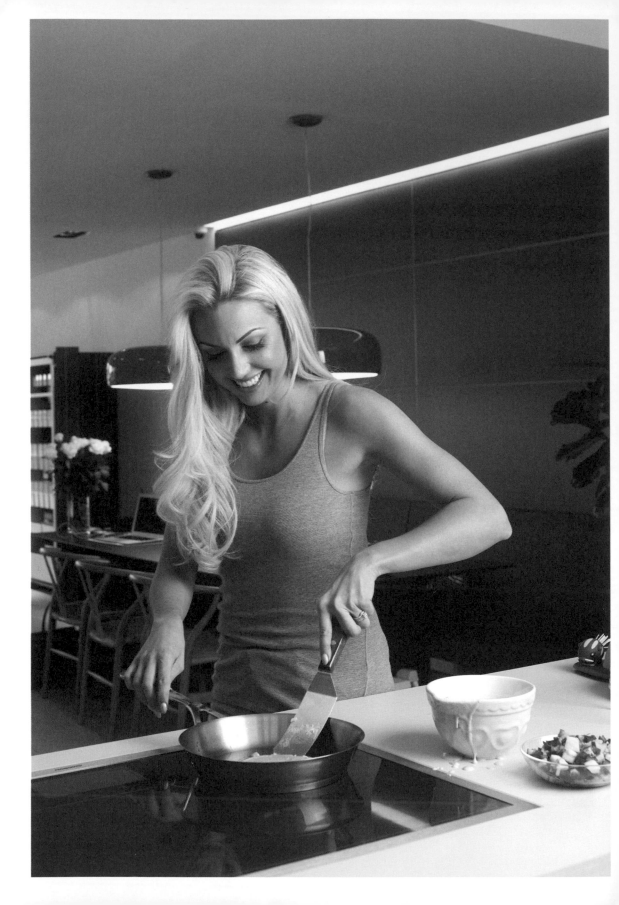

SAVOURY BUCKWHEAT PANCAKE WRAPS WITH SPICY PINEAPPLE SALSA

Makes 10 pancakes

330g buckwheat flour

pinch of Himalayan pink rock salt

750ml + 2 tbsp cold water

1 tbsp ground flaxseed

1 tbsp coconut oil

FOR THE TOPPINGS:

spicy pineapple salsa (page 146)

zesty guacamole (page 153)

handful of rocket

This dish ended up being the happy result of some experimentation in the kitchen. I love to make a spicy pineapple salsa to add a twist to veggies and quinoa dishes, and I was planning a savoury version of buckwheat pancakes to have for dinner. I simply piled the salsa onto the pancakes with some crisp fresh rocket leaves and a dollop of my zesty guacamole and then made them into wraps for a really fresh, satisfying and vibrantly coloured meal.

1   Mix the flour and a pinch of salt in a large bowl. Make a well in the centre of the flour and slowly pour in 750ml water, whisking continuously to ensure the batter is smooth.

2   In a separate small bowl, mix together the ground flaxseed and 2 tablespoons of water to make the flaxseed 'egg'. Add this to the batter in the large bowl and mix well.

3   Heat the coconut oil in a frying pan until it bubbles and pour in a ladleful of the batter. Cook for a few minutes, until the bottom of the pancake has set and browned, then flip over and cook the other side for a few minutes more, until browned.

4   Serve with the savoury toppings. I make large, thin pancakes for wraps but they can also be made small and thick if preferred.

DIPS AND DRESSINGS

These are my favourite healthy salad dressings and dips to encourage you to focus on your eating plan with plenty of salads, raw vegetables and wraps. I've included a range of different flavours, herbs and spices to jazz up even the most simple salads and crudités. They're all easy to whizz up in a blender and are all bursting with the nutrients you need to reach your highest health and beauty potential.

Beauty tip:

AIM TO INCORPORATE **FRAGRANT HERBS** LIKE PARSLEY, CORIANDER, MINT, BASIL, ROSEMARY AND SAGE INTO YOUR REGULAR DIET TO BENEFIT FROM THEIR DETOXING AND SKIN-BRIGHTENING PROPERTIES. SPICES ARE ALSO A GREAT WAY TO BOOST THE FLAVOUR OF MEALS WITHOUT USING UNHEALTHY SALT, SUGAR AND OILS. I LOVE SMOKED PAPRIKA, CURRY POWDER, TURMERIC, CAYENNE PEPPER, CHILLI, GINGER AND CUMIN.

ROSIE'S CLASSIC SALAD DRESSING

Serves 2

2 ripe, medium tomatoes

1 clove of garlic, peeled

juice of $1/2$ lemon or lime

2 heaped tbsp nutritional yeast

2 heaped tbsp hulled hemp seeds

2 tbsp raw apple cider vinegar

2 tbsp Coconut Aminos, Bragg Liquid Amino or low-sodium tamari sauce

$1/2$ tsp smoked paprika

Rosie is my nickname and this is my favourite dressing to whizz up and pour over a marinated kale and avocado salad (page 109). It's one of my go-to quick and nourishing weekday meals and it's so easy to prepare. I adore the combination of flavours, and a tasty salad dressing can really help to make salads and veggies the main part of your evening meal. This tangy dressing offers a good balance of 17g of high-fibre plant protein from the hemp seeds and nutritional yeast; B vitamins, zinc, iron, omega-3 fats, vitamin C and antioxidants from the tomatoes; probiotic benefits from the raw apple cider vinegar; and the antifungal and antibacterial properties of the garlic.

1   Place all the ingredients in a food processor or blender and blend until smooth. Pour generously over your salad.
2   Store the dressing in an airtight container or screw-top jar in the fridge for up to three days.

CITRUS TAHINI DRESSING

Serves 2–3

juice of 1 large orange

juice of 1 lemon

1 clove of garlic, peeled

2 tbsp tahini

1 tbsp apple cider vinegar

1 tsp roughly chopped fresh ginger

3–4 drops of liquid stevia or 1 tsp raw local honey (optional)

Himalayan pink rock salt and freshly ground black pepper

I'm a big fan of tahini as it's so versatile and nourishing. This is yet another way to enjoy it drizzled over salads, sushi and as a raw vegetable dip. It's thick, creamy and full of flavour yet free from the unhealthy oils, sugar and preservatives in shop-bought dressings.

1. Place all the ingredients in a blender and combine until smooth. Taste and add a little extra seasoning or sweetener if necessary.
2. Store the dressing in an airtight container or screw-top jar in the fridge for up to three days.

GINGER SESAME DRESSING

Serves 2–3

1 clove of garlic, peeled

3 tbsp tahini

1 tbsp finely chopped fresh ginger

1 tbsp low-sodium tamari

1 tbsp pure maple syrup

2 tsp rice wine vinegar

1 tsp Dijon mustard

1 tsp sesame seeds, to garnish

I love the fresh, tangy flavours of this dressing. It really brightens up a raw, crunchy salad and works well as a dip for raw veggies when a healthy snack is required. Sesame seeds are a good source of calcium, while warming ginger boosts digestion and supports your immune system.

1. Place all the ingredients in a blender and blend until smooth. Add a little water if the dressing is too thick.
2. Pour into a serving bowl and garnish with the sesame seeds.
3. Store the dressing in an airtight container or screw-top jar in the fridge for up to three days.

CREAMY AVOCADO DRESSING

Serves 2

1 ripe avocado, peeled and pitted

2 cloves of garlic, peeled

2 tbsp freshly squeezed lemon juice

2 tbsp finely diced red onion

1 tsp smoked paprika

pinch of cayenne pepper

Himalayan pink rock salt and freshly ground black pepper

Avocado is one of the very best healthy fats for youthful skin and shiny hair, so this dressing is a little piece of heaven for your complexion and your taste buds. Avocado blends into the most deliciously thick and creamy texture, perfect for drizzling over salads or using as a dip for raw veggie sticks.

1 Place all the ingredients in a blender and combine together until the dressing is a thick liquid consistency.

2 Store the dressing in an airtight container or screw-top jar in the fridge for up to three days.

SKIN-BRIGHTENING SMOKY SWEET PEPPER AND WALNUT DIP

Serves 2–3

180g walnuts, chopped

2 large red peppers, halved and deseeded

1 clove of garlic, chopped

120ml unsweetened almond milk

1 tsp smoked paprika

squeeze of fresh lime juice

pinch of cayenne pepper (optional)

Himalayan pink rock salt and freshly ground black pepper

I simply had to refer to the incredible skin benefits in the title of this raw dip, as it contains two of the very best foods for fresher, younger-looking and plumper skin: walnuts and red pepper.
It's always a big hit in my house, as my husband loves its smoky flavour and creamy texture. I eat it with raw veggies and energy crackers, dolloped onto salads or as a base in cabbage tacos and nori wraps. I usually make a big enough batch to store in the fridge and eat over a few days.

1   Soak the walnuts in a bowl of cold water for 3–4 hours. Drain and rinse well.
2   Add all the ingredients to a blender. Blend on a high speed until the mixture is smooth. Add a little extra almond milk if necessary to help it blend.
3   Store any leftover dip in an airtight container or screw-top jar in the fridge for up to three days.

ROASTED RED PEPPER AND CORIANDER HUMMUS

Serves 2

1 red pepper

200g cooked chickpeas (see page 22 for cooking instructions)

1 clove of garlic, peeled

juice of $\frac{1}{2}$ lemon

3 tbsp chopped fresh coriander

2 tbsp tahini

1 tsp ground cumin

1 tsp smoked paprika

Himalayan pink rock salt and freshly ground black pepper

This is such a simple and quick snack or meal component, rich in protein and healthy fats. I always keep tahini and chickpeas in the cupboard so that I can whip up this hummus to eat with alkalising raw veggie sticks or paired with fresh rocket on an open wheat-free toasted sandwich. I love the extra flavour that the roasted red pepper, coriander and spices bring to it, plus they're some of the best foods for glowing skin and a healthy body.

1 Preheat the oven to 200°C.
2 Place the red pepper on a small baking tray and roast in the oven for about 20 minutes, until it's slightly charred on the outside. Cut in half and remove the seeds.
3 Add the pepper and the remaining ingredients to a blender or food processor and blend until the hummus is almost smooth. I like to leave a few chunks for texture, but add a little water if you prefer it smoother.
4 Store the hummus in an airtight container or screw-top jar in the fridge for up to three days.

LIVER DETOX LEMON AND PARSLEY HUMMUS

Serves 2

200g cooked chickpeas (see page 22 for cooking instructions)

20g fresh parsley, long stems removed and leaves chopped, plus 1 sprig to garnish

1 clove of garlic, peeled

2 tbsp freshly squeezed lemon juice

2 tbsp tahini

1 tbsp extra virgin olive oil

$1/2$ tsp ground cumin

pinch of dried chilli flakes

Himalayan pink rock salt and freshly ground black pepper

pinch of smoked paprika, to garnish

Your liver is an important organ for your health and beauty, and a congested liver is associated with an array of health and beauty issues, such as acne. One of my areas of focus when working with clients is ensuring that their liver is fortified by their diet and lifestyle choices. An optimally functioning liver will really help you to reach your health and wellness goals. Parsley and lemon are both powerful foods for supporting normal liver detoxification and helping it to remove any toxic build-up from your body.

1 Place all the ingredients in a blender and combine until the hummus is creamy and smooth. Add a little water if you prefer it less thick.

2 Spoon the hummus into a serving bowl. Garnish with a sprig of parsley and a sprinkle of smoked paprika.

3 Store the hummus in an airtight container or screw-top jar in the fridge for up to three days.

SPICY PINEAPPLE SALSA

Serves 2

250g fresh pineapple, finely diced

100g cucumber, deseeded and finely diced

1 red pepper, deseeded and finely diced

1/2 large red onion, finely diced

3 tbsp finely chopped fresh coriander

3 tbsp freshly squeezed lime juice

2 tbsp finely diced jalapeño

Himalayan pink rock salt and freshly ground black pepper

This is another Mauritian-inspired dish that is often served at our favourite hotel on their Mauritian buffet night. I always end up spooning a pile of it onto the side of my plate, as it seems to go with everything. I love the contrast of sweet, juicy pineapple with the coriander, crunchy peppers, cucumber and spicy jalapeño. Pineapple is also an excellent food for stimulating your digestive enzymes, so try to eat this salsa with a starter course to get the most health benefits.

1   Combine all the ingredients in a mixing bowl. Season to taste with salt and pepper. Mix well and allow to sit for 10–15 minutes to let the flavours develop. Serve immediately or keep refrigerated until ready to serve.

2   If making the salsa ahead of time, it can be stored in an airtight container in the fridge for up to three days.

CREAMY GARLIC
AND LIME PEA PURÉE

SPICY
PINEAPPLE SALSA

SKIN-BRIGHTENING
SMOKY SWEET PEPPER
AND WALNUT DIP

CLASSIC TOMATO SALSA

Serves 3–4

6 ripe plum tomatoes

¹/₂ red onion, finely diced

2 cloves of garlic, minced

1 serrano chilli, finely diced
(remove the seeds for
less heat)

8 tbsp finely chopped
fresh coriander

2 tbsp freshly squeezed
lime juice

1 tbsp balsamic vinegar

1 tsp low-sodium tamari

Himalayan pink rock salt and
freshly ground black pepper

A consistently popular dip for sweet potato wedges, crackers and veggie sticks, this classic tomato salsa also works well as a healthy and simple low-calorie salad dressing. I make a big batch every few days and keep it refrigerated in an airtight container, as it always gets used up quickly in my house. It's also a great way to get kids to eat their vegetables. Tomatoes are packed with lycopene, a powerful carotenoid antioxidant. Furthermore, the humble tomato is rich in collagen-building vitamin C for firm, smooth skin and biotin for healthy hair growth.

1 Cut the tomatoes in half to remove their seeds and core. Chop the flesh into small pieces.
2 Place the tomatoes in a mixing bowl with the rest of the ingredients. Mix well and allow to sit for 10–15 minutes to let the flavours develop. Serve immediately or keep refrigerated until ready to serve.
3 If making the salsa ahead of time, it can be stored in an airtight container in the fridge for up to three days.

VEGAN BASIL PESTO

Makes 2 servings

135g pine nuts

45g fresh basil leaves, rinsed well

4 cloves of garlic, peeled

4 heaped tbsp nutritional yeast

2 tbsp cold-pressed extra virgin olive oil

2 tbsp freshly squeezed lemon juice

2 tbsp unsweetened almond milk

Himalayan pink rock salt and freshly ground black pepper

Pesto works so well with a wide range of salads, wraps and main dishes, but I tend to make it most often to accompany my raw courgetti (page 164) and rainbow glow bowl (page 114), as it complements the simple veggies so well. To make a lower-fat version of the classic recipe, I've replaced some of the quantities of olive oil traditionally used with almond milk.

1 Mix all the ingredients in a blender or food processor until the pine nuts are ground down, but ensure some texture remains and the pesto isn't entirely smooth. Taste and add more garlic, lemon juice or seasoning if required.

2 Transfer to an airtight container or a screw-top jar. Covered with a thin film of olive oil and kept in the fridge, the pesto will keep for up to three days.

CREAMY GARLIC, AND LIME PEA PURÉE

Serves 3–4

220g steamed peas

3 cloves of garlic, peeled

juice of 2 limes

2 tbsp nutritional yeast

Himalayan pink rock salt and freshly ground black pepper

splash of unsweetened almond milk, to blend (optional)

I've been making this dish each Christmas for my family for the past few years, as well as plenty of other times throughout the year. Everyone loves the contrast of the vibrant green colour and tangy flavour with the heavy festive foods. I often make it to accompany roast vegetables, quinoa and veggie curries and even big salads, as the naturally smooth and creamy texture of the purée works well as a dip or dressing. The peas also pack a good protein punch, plus plenty of fibre to keep your digestive system in optimal health.

1   Place all the ingredients in a blender or food processor and blend at a high speed until smooth and creamy. Use a little almond milk to help it blend if required.
2   Store the purée in an airtight container in the fridge for up to three days.

MINTY COCONUT CHUTNEY

Serves 2

40g fresh coriander, washed and trimmed

120ml low-fat coconut milk

juice of $\frac{1}{2}$ lemon

2 tbsp fresh mint leaves

2 tbsp unsweetened coconut flakes

pinch of cayenne pepper

Himalayan pink rock salt and freshly ground black pepper

I love this fresh minty chutney on top of salads and in wraps with a few chunks of avocado. It also works a treat with my veggie burgers (page 182) and baked falafels (page 171).

1   Whizz all the ingredients together in a blender, adding a little more coconut milk if a thinner consistency is required.
2   Store the chutney in an airtight container or screw-top jar in the fridge for up to three days.

MOROCCAN-SPICED CARROT GUACAMOLE

Serves 2

3 large carrots, peeled and chopped into chunks

250ml coconut milk

$1/2$ tsp curry powder

1 ripe avocado, pitted, peeled and sliced

1 clove of garlic, peeled

juice of $1/2$ lemon

1 tbsp tahini

$1/2$ tsp smoked paprika

$1/2$ tsp ground turmeric

$1/2$ tsp ground coriander

$1/2$ tsp ground cumin

pinch of dried chilli flakes

Himalayan pink rock salt and freshly ground black pepper

I'm a big fan of homemade dips, as there are so many flavour options to choose from. All you need is a bit of imagination! I decided to create a guacamole-style carrot dip and add in a variety of Moroccan spices to accompany dishes like the baked falafels on page 171. It's easy to whip up for visiting friends and family, plus it makes a tasty and nutritious lunch. The tahini (sesame seed paste) and avocado help to boost its levels of calcium, iron, potassium, healthy fats and protein.

1   In a small saucepan over a medium heat, simmer the chopped carrots in the coconut milk with the curry powder for 8–10 minutes, until soft.

2   Pour the carrots and coconut milk into a blender with the rest of the ingredients. Blend together until the guacamole is smooth and creamy.

3   Store the guacamole in an airtight container in the fridge for up to three days.

SKIN-QUENCHING ZESTY GUACAMOLE

Serves 2

1 ripe avocado
1 medium tomato
1 clove of garlic, peeled
juice of 1 lemon
$1/2$ tsp smoked paprika
a pinch of cayenne pepper
Himalayan pink rock salt and freshly ground black pepper

Avocado is one of the very best foods for building smooth, firm, plump skin. It quenches dehydrated skin with plenty of essential fatty acids, while the vitamin C in the lemon helps collagen to form for a younger-looking complexion. Eat up!

1 Cut the avocado in half lengthways and remove the stone. Scoop the soft flesh into a blender or food processor, followed by the rest of the ingredients. Blend until well combined, but leave some chunks if you prefer more texture. If you don't have a blender, mash the avocado with a fork, finely chop the tomato and crush the garlic and mix together along with the rest of the ingredients.
2 Store the guacamole in an airtight container in the fridge for up to three days.

RECIPES

MAIN DISHES

Many of these main dishes are packed with warming and
nourishing cooked plant foods to satisfy hungry tummies and
big appetites. My own meat-eating husband loves many of these
meals, as they leave him feeling well-fed and full for hours.
Cooked foods also help you to get through chilly winter months
when you crave more sustenance, but eating plenty of raw foods
is also important to benefit from their beauty- and health-
enhancing living enzymes. You should always aim to accompany
cooked meals with lots of green salads and raw veggies.

Beauty tip:

GET USED TO EATING UNTIL YOU'RE
THREE-QUARTERS FULL. IT CAN BE
TEMPTING TO EAT EVERY SINGLE BITE
ON YOUR PLATE, BUT PORTIONS TODAY
ARE OFTEN VERY BIG. YOU SHOULD FEEL
LIGHT AND ENERGISED AFTER A MEAL,
NOT BLOATED, HEAVY AND TIRED. TRY
USING A SIDE PLATE INSTEAD OF A DINNER
PLATE, AS SMALLER PORTIONS WILL MAKE
ALL THE DIFFERENCE TO HEALTHY AND
SUSTAINABLE WEIGHT LOSS. ONE OF MY
FAVOURITE TRICKS IS TO FILL UP ON A BIG
GREEN SALAD DRESSED WITH LEMON JUICE
AND RAW APPLE CIDER VINEGAR BEFORE
MOVING ON TO THE REST OF THE MEAL.

LENTIL, SWEET POTATO AND RED PEPPER BAKED LOAF

Makes 1 loaf

400g green lentils

1 tbsp ground flaxseed

2 tbsp water

$^1/_2$ tbsp coconut oil, plus extra for greasing

150g red pepper, diced

1 red onion, finely diced

2 cloves of garlic, minced

Himalayan pink rock salt and freshly ground black pepper

1 medium sweet potato, finely chopped or shredded

250g tomato passata (I use an organic brand sold in glass jars rather than cans)

75g gluten-free rolled oats

30g fresh flat-leaf parsley, chopped

1 tbsp chopped fresh rosemary

1 tbsp dried thyme

2 tsp smoked paprika, plus a pinch to garnish

This is one of my favourite plant-based dishes to make for Christmas Day, as the red and green of the peppers and coriander make it look suitably festive. It's a satisfying dish thanks to the protein- and fibre-packed lentils and complexion-nourishing sweet potato, while the parsley, onion and garlic help to support liver detoxification. As it's a cooked dish, I love to eat it with a big green salad and plenty of raw veggies for optimal digestion.

1   To cook the lentils, first rinse them in a sieve under cold running water. Transfer them to a medium saucepan and cover with double their volume of water. Over a medium-high heat, bring the lentils to a rapid simmer and then reduce the temperature to gently simmer them, uncovered, for 20–30 minutes. The lentils should be just barely covered with water and are cooked once they're tender rather than crunchy.

2   Preheat the oven to 180°C. Lightly grease a loaf tin with coconut oil.

3   Prepare the flax 'egg' by placing the ground flaxseed in a small bowl and mixing with the water. Place in the fridge to set for 10 minutes.

4   Heat the coconut oil in a frying pan over a medium heat. Cook the diced peppers, onion and garlic for 6–7 minutes, until soft and lightly browned. Add salt and pepper to taste.

5   In a large mixing bowl, combine the cooked lentils, flax 'egg', sweet potato, passata, oats, parsley, rosemary, thyme and smoked paprika plus more seasoning if desired. Add the red pepper mixture and stir until everything is mixed well.

6   Pour the mixture into the greased loaf tin and ensure it's smooth and even. Sprinkle with another pinch of smoked paprika.

7   Bake for 45–50 minutes, until the loaf is firm to touch and brown on top.

8   Remove from the oven and transfer to a cooling rack. Slice into individual portions and serve warm or cold. Store in an airtight container in the fridge for up to four days.

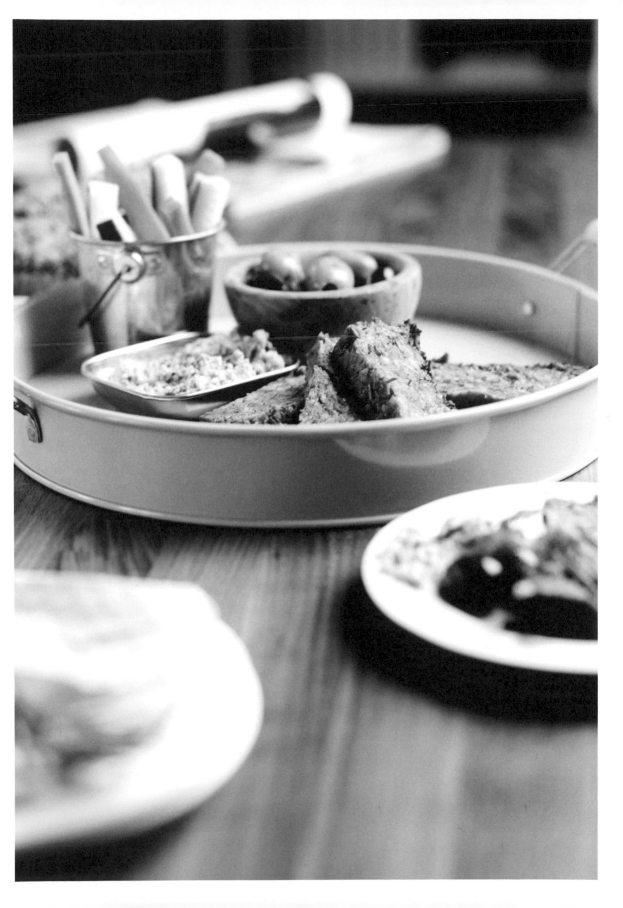

ANTI-INFLAMMATORY TURMERIC AND MAPLE ROASTED CAULIFLOWER, CARROT AND SWEET POTATO

Serves 2

1 tbsp pure organic maple syrup

1 tbsp coconut oil, melted

1 tbsp ground turmeric

2 medium carrots, peeled and cut into chunks

1 head of cauliflower, broken into florets

1 medium sweet potato, unpeeled and cut into wedges

Himalayan pink rock salt and freshly ground black pepper

2 tbsp toasted sesame seeds, to garnish

3 tbsp chopped fresh coriander, to garnish

1 tbsp finely grated fresh ginger, to garnish

This wholesome and comforting roast vegetable dish combines some of the very best ingredients for your immune system to help your body fight off pesky bugs and viruses. Turmeric and ginger are two of the best spices for improving digestion, reducing inflammation throughout the body and warming you up on cold days. Cauliflower, carrots and sweet potatoes are a great combination to fill up a hungry tummy with fibre and essential nutrients. I like to pair this dish with a big green salad for dinner.

1 Preheat the oven to 190°C.
2 Mix together the maple syrup, melted coconut oil and turmeric in a small bowl.
3 Put the chopped vegetables onto a large baking tray. Pour over the maple mixture until the vegetables are coated well. Season with salt and pepper.
4 Roast in the oven for 35-40 minutes, until the vegetables are lightly browned and softened.
5 Meanwhile, lightly toast the sesame seeds in a small, dry pan over a medium heat just until they start to turn golden. Take care not to burn them.
6 Transfer the vegetables to a serving platter and garnish with the toasted sesame seeds, coriander and grated ginger.

ROAST BUTTERNUT SQUASH AND CHICKPEA STEW

Serves 3–4

1 butternut squash, washed and left whole

1 low-sodium vegetable stock cube

500ml boiling water

1 tsp organic virgin coconut oil, plus extra for greasing

2 large red peppers, chopped into bite-sized chunks

1 red onion, chopped into bite-sized chunks

70g mushrooms, chopped into bite-sized chunks

1 clove of garlic, chopped

200g cooked chickpeas (see page 22 for cooking instructions)

1 tsp ground cumin

1 tsp ground turmeric

1 tsp curry powder

120ml coconut milk

Himalayan pink rock salt and freshly ground black pepper

2–3 handfuls of baby spinach leaves

1 tbsp pumpkin seeds, to garnish

This is a deliciously warming, nourishing and easy dish to whip up. It's also a cheap and filling option for families, students and anyone watching the pennies, plus kids will love the natural sweetness of the butternut squash and peppers. Beta-carotene, which gives the squash and peppers their vibrant colour, is especially important for bright, healthy eyes, good vision and glowing skin. I add in chickpeas and spinach for a healthy boost of plant protein. The chopped mushrooms give it a meatier texture, and onion and garlic have sulphur-containing nutrients to support liver function. This stew is great on its own or served with quinoa or brown rice.

1 Preheat the oven to 200°C. Lightly grease a baking tray with coconut oil.

2 Place the butternut squash on the greased baking tray. Roast the whole squash for 20–25 minutes, until softened and slightly browned on the outside. When it's cool enough to handle, cut in half and remove the seeds, remove the skin and then chop the flesh into chunks.

3 Meanwhile, dissolve the vegetable stock cube in the boiling water.

4 Heat the coconut oil in a saucepan on a medium heat. Sauté the peppers, onion, mushrooms and garlic for 4–5 minutes, until the vegetables are starting to soften.

5 Add the cooked chickpeas, chopped squash and vegetable stock and bring to a boil on a medium-high heat before partly covering with a lid and reducing to a simmer. Add the spices and coconut milk. Taste it and adapt the seasoning to your own preference. Stir occasionally for 10–15 minutes, until the water has evaporated and a thick stew has formed. Remove from the heat, stir in the baby spinach leaves and allow them to wilt.

6 Ladle into bowls and sprinkle with pumpkin seeds just before serving.

COCONUT CURRY WITH SWEET POTATO NOODLES

Serves 2–3

FOR THE COCONUT CURRY:

1 tbsp organic virgin coconut oil

50g cauliflower florets

50g broccoli florets

2 large carrots, peeled and diced

1/2 medium red onion, diced

2 cloves of garlic, minced

Himalayan pink rock salt and freshly ground black pepper

250ml low-sodium vegetable stock

250ml low-fat coconut milk

1 serrano chilli, finely diced (remove the seeds for less heat)

1 tbsp curry powder

1 tsp ground cumin

50g sugar snap peas, each one cut in half

1 ripe plum tomato, chopped

2 tbsp chopped fresh coriander, to garnish

FOR THE SWEET POTATO NOODLES:

3 medium sweet potatoes, peeled

1 tbsp organic virgin coconut oil

1/2 medium red onion, diced

2 cloves of garlic, minced

1 tbsp grated fresh ginger

1 tsp smoked paprika

pinch of dried chilli flakes

Himalayan pink rock salt and freshly ground black pepper

This snazzy little dish ticks all the boxes for a simple, warming and fibre-rich meal. Plus substituting regular wheat-based noodles for sweet potato noodles means you won't end up in a digestive slump afterwards, spending precious energy trying to process the sticky gluten. As a slow-release complex carb, the sweet potato will sustain your energy levels and impart all of its skin-brightening beta-carotene benefits.

1 First make the noodles. Using a spiraliser or vegetable peeler, cut the peeled sweet potatoes into long strips to resemble noodles.

2 Heat the coconut oil in a large saucepan or skillet over a medium heat. Sauté the onion, garlic and ginger for 5 minutes, until slightly browned. Add the sweet potato noodles and sauté for about 5 minutes, until they soften. Add 1 or 2 tablespoons of water if they start to look too dry. Add the smoked paprika and dried chilli flakes and season to taste. Remove from the heat, cover and set aside while you make the coconut curry.

3 Heat the coconut oil in a large saucepan over a medium heat. Sauté the cauliflower, broccoli, carrots, onion and garlic for 8–10 minutes, stirring often, until the vegetables have softened. Season to taste.

4 Add in the vegetable stock, coconut milk, diced chilli, curry powder and cumin. Bring to the boil over a medium-high heat, then cover partly with a lid, reduce the heat and simmer for 12–15 minutes, until slightly reduced.

5 Add in the sugar snap peas and chopped tomatoes and stir well. Remove from the heat and season again if desired.

6 Divide the sweet potato noodles between two or three plates. Spoon the coconut curry over the noodles and garnish with the fresh coriander.

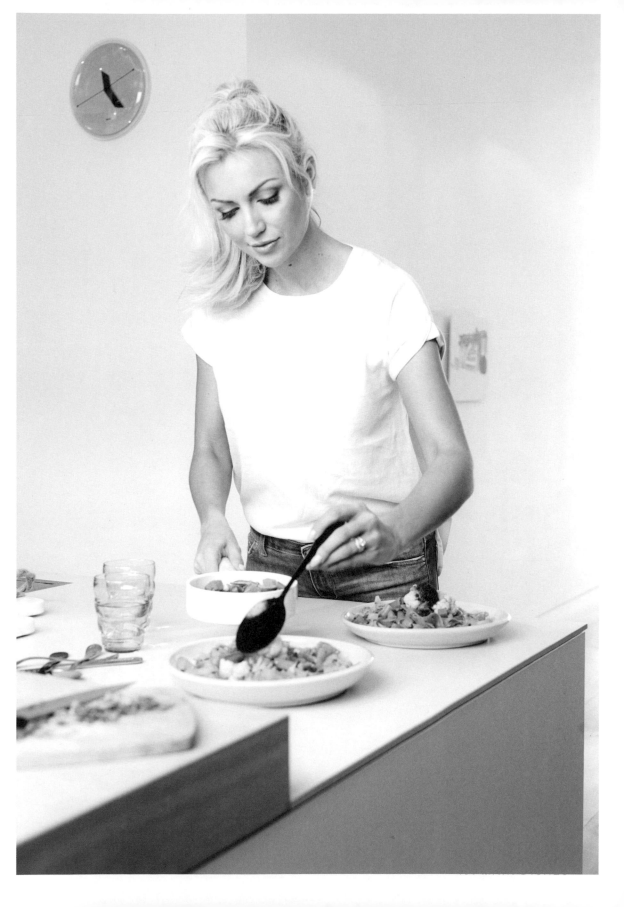

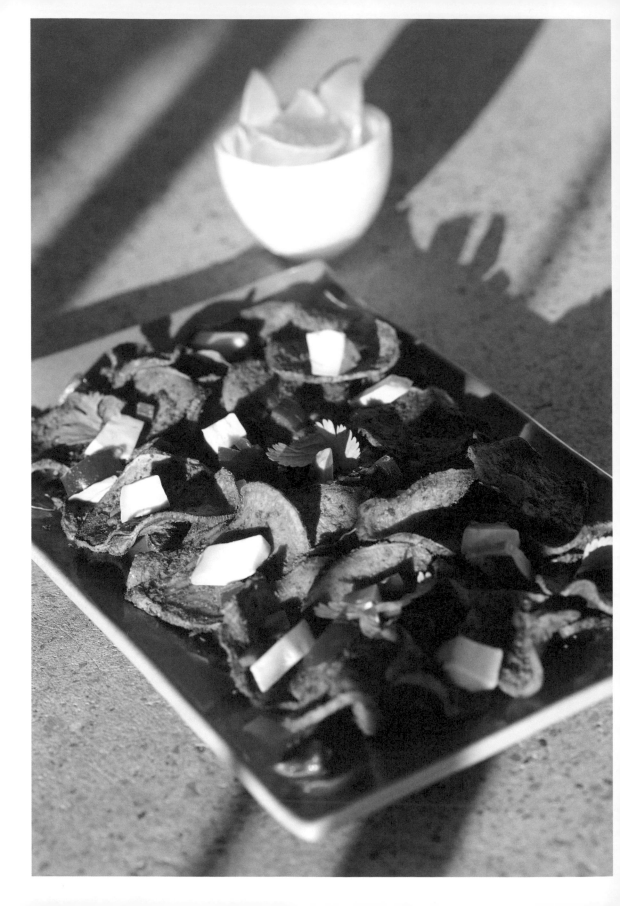

LOADED SWEET POTATO NACHOS WITH ZESTY GUACAMOLE

Serves 2

2 medium sweet potatoes

1 tbsp coconut oil, melted

1 tsp curry powder

1 tsp ground turmeric

1 tsp smoked paprika

Himalayan pink rock salt and freshly ground black pepper

2 tbsp nutritional yeast

zesty guacamole (page 153),

½ ripe avocado, diced (optional)

cherry tomatoes, halved

chopped jalapeños

Nachos! They're usually just an occasional treat for most people, as they aren't exactly waistline friendly. This version of nachos, however, is highly nutritious for your skin and body. The sweet potato caramelises in the oven, becoming chewy with crispy edges, while the zesty guacamole adds a delicious twist. Sweet potatoes are a true superstar root vegetable and a good complex carbohydrate to enjoy in your diet frequently. They're also a great source of beta-carotene, which is important for eye and skin health and for a glowing complexion. They contain fibre, potassium, calcium and magnesium, plus vitamin C necessary for collagen production in the skin and vitamin B6 to boost your mood. They're a true feel-good food for health and beauty.

1   Preheat the oven to 200°C. Line a baking tray with grease-proof paper.
2   Scrub the sweet potatoes well. I like to leave the skin on to go crispy in the oven. Slice the potatoes as thinly as possible with a sharp serrated knife.
3   In a small bowl, mix together the melted coconut oil with the curry powder, turmeric, smoked paprika and some salt and pepper.
4   Toss the sweet potato slices in the spice mixture, coating them well. Lay them out on the lined baking tray and sprinkle with the nutritional yeast.
5   Bake in the oven for 20–25 minutes, until they become crispy around the edges.
6   Arrange the nachos on a serving platter with a dollop of guacamole and scatter with the avocado, cherry tomatoes and chopped jalapeños.

RAW COURGETTI WITH SUN-DRIED TOMATO PESTO

Serves 2

2 medium courgettes,
topped and tailed

2 tbsp freshly squeezed
lemon juice

Himalayan pink rock salt and
freshly ground black pepper

6 cherry tomatoes, halved

1 ripe avocado, pitted,
peeled and sliced

2 tbsp chopped fresh basil

1 tbsp nutritional yeast

FOR THE SUN-DRIED TOMATO PESTO:

80g sun-dried tomatoes

50g pine nuts

2 cloves of garlic, chopped

2 heaped tbsp nutritional yeast

2 tbsp cold-pressed extra
virgin olive oil

2 tbsp unsweetened
almond milk

Himalayan pink rock salt and
freshly ground black pepper

Courgetti is simply raw courgette that has been put through a spiraliser so that it resembles spaghetti. It has all of the texture and versatility of the popular Italian dish, but none of the gluten. As much as I like the idea of digging into a huge plate of steaming hot spaghetti, I know that my digestion would seriously suffer for it, and encouraging optimal digestion is the ultimate secret to vibrant beauty and health. This is one of my favourite easy, raw, inexpensive and satisfying meals to put together when time is limited.

1   To make the pesto, place all the ingredients in a blender and combine until almost smooth, scraping down the sides when necessary.

2   Process the courgettes through a spiraliser to create the raw courgetti. A vegetable peeler can also be used to slice the courgettes into ribbons. Place in a large mixing bowl and drizzle with the lemon juice. Season to taste and toss well.

3   Pile the courgetti onto two serving plates. Top with a dollop of the sun-dried tomato pesto, cherry tomatoes, sliced avocado, fresh basil and a sprinkle of nutritional yeast and serve.

4   Transfer any leftover pesto to an airtight container or a screw-top jar. Covered with a thin film of olive oil and kept in the fridge, the pesto will keep for up to four days.

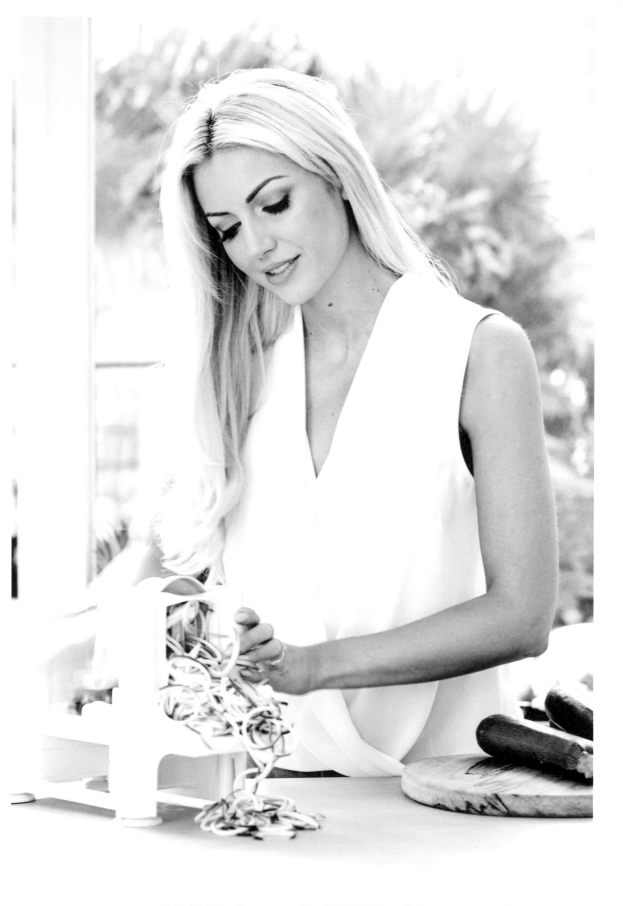

PROTEIN PUNCH
PIZZA

Makes 1 pizza

130g quinoa

60ml water

1 tsp gluten-free baking powder

1 tsp dried oregano

1 tsp ground turmeric

pinch of Himalayan pink rock salt

1 tbsp organic virgin coconut oil, melted

Growing up, pizza was a much-anticipated Friday night treat. We lived within walking distance of a great pizzeria, and even as a child I would always order the vegetarian pizza. I loved toppings like peppers, pineapple and sweetcorn, though the pizza was thickly covered with a hot layer of melted mozzarella. Luckily, I have found an excellent alternative in quinoa as a protein-packed pizza base infused with a little anti-inflammatory turmeric and antibacterial oregano. Simply top the base with your favourite flavours. I love a hearty raw vegan pesto (page 149) topped with chilli-lime avocado (page 96), rocket and cherry tomatoes drizzled with lime juice, a pinch of chilli flakes and some salt and pepper.

1   Preheat the oven to 220°C. Line a 20cm springform cake tin with greaseproof paper.
2   Rinse the quinoa well in a sieve. Place it in a food processor or blender with the water, baking powder, oregano, turmeric and a pinch of salt. Blend until smooth.
3   Pour the melted coconut oil on top of the paper in the lined tin. Pour the pizza base mixture onto the greased paper, using a spatula to ensure it's flat and even.
4   Bake in the oven for 15 minutes. Remove from the oven, carefully turn the pizza base over and bake the other side for 5–10 minutes more, until it's firm and golden brown.
5   Remove the pizza base from the oven and turn it out onto a wire rack to allow it to cool slightly and crisp up before adding your toppings. Serve warm or cold.

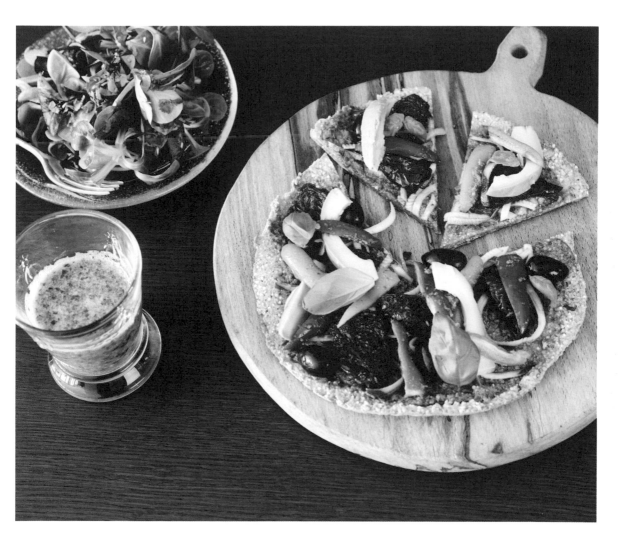

SLEEPYTIME SWEET POTATO AND MILLET BURGERS WITH CARAMELISED RED ONION AND FENNEL RELISH

Makes 8 burgers

200g millet

500ml water

1 tsp coconut oil, for greasing

4 medium sweet potatoes, peeled

360g baby spinach

60g buckwheat flour

2 cloves of garlic, minced

2 tbsp ground flaxseed

1 tsp smoked paprika

1 tsp ground turmeric

1 tsp ground cumin

pinch of crushed dried chilli flakes

Himalayan pink rock salt and freshly ground black pepper

60ml unsweetened almond milk (optional)

chilli-lime avocado (page 96), to serve

FOR THE CARAMELISED RED ONION AND FENNEL RELISH:

4 tbsp balsamic vinegar

1 tsp coconut palm sugar

1 red onion, thinly sliced

1 tsp fennel seeds

Himalayan pink rock salt and freshly ground black pepper

Millet may look a little like bird food, but it's a great alternative to other nutrient-packed grains like quinoa. It's a super source of copper, phosphorus, manganese and magnesium. Magnesium is nature's own sedative, helping to relax your muscles, lower your blood pressure and make you feel calm and clear. That means a healthier heart, less chance of stress-related headaches and migraines, and better quality of sleep. Sweet potatoes are also a dream for poor sleepers due to their levels of tryptophan, which helps to produce the sleep hormone, serotonin. I've popped in the spinach for an extra serving of greens, plus smoked paprika and cumin for their warming flavours. These delicious burgers make a great dinner served with a salad and piled high with my caramelised red onion and fennel relish and chilli-lime avocado.

1   To cook the millet, rinse it well in a sieve. Place the water in a saucepan, add in the millet and bring to the boil over a medium-high heat. Reduce the heat, cover partly with a lid and simmer for 10–15 minutes, until the millet seeds have swollen and the water has almost boiled off. Remove from the heat and allow the remaining bit of water to be absorbed.

2   Preheat the oven to 200°C. Lightly grease two baking trays with the teaspoon of coconut oil.

3   Scrub two of the sweet potatoes, chop them into bite-sized chunks and steam just until soft. Rinse the baby spinach and lightly steam until it has just wilted.

4   Place the steamed sweet potatoes and spinach in a blender or food processor. Add the cooked millet and the remaining burger ingredients and blend to combine. Add a splash of almond milk if the mixture is too dry to stick together.

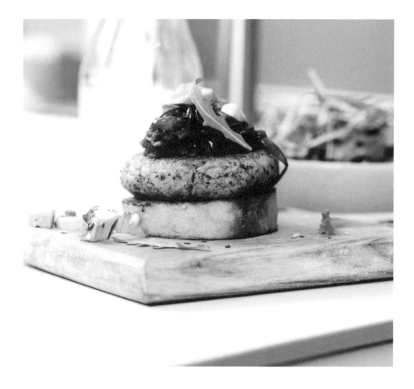

5 Roll up your sleeves and use your hands to form the mixture into eight burgers. Each one should be about 1.25cm thick and 10cm in diameter. Place on one of the greased baking trays.

6 Cook the burgers in the oven for 35–40 minutes, flipping them over after 15–20 minutes to allow both sides to turn golden brown.

7 Cut the two remaining sweet potatoes into slices about 1.25cm thick and place on the second greased baking tray. Season with a pinch of salt and pepper and bake in the oven alongside the burgers for approximately 30 minutes, until golden brown and crisp around the edges. Remove from the oven and set aside until you're ready to serve.

8 Meanwhile, to make the relish, gently heat the balsamic vinegar and coconut palm sugar in a small saucepan over a medium heat. Add the red onion and cook for 4–5 minutes, until it begins to soften. Add the fennel seeds and seasoning and continue to cook for another 2–3 minutes, until it caramelises. Take care not to let it burn. Add a splash of boiled water if it appears too dry. Remove from the heat and allow to cool for 10 minutes.

9 Put the sweet potato burger 'buns' on serving plates and top with the burgers, some caramelised red onion relish and chilli-lime avocado.

ALKALISING ROAST MILLET PEPPERS

Serves 3–4

175g millet

450ml water

1 tbsp organic virgin coconut oil, plus extra for greasing

1/2 large red onion, diced

2 cloves of garlic, minced

1 large carrot, peeled and chopped

70g raw kale, chopped

40g unsalted walnuts, chopped

30g fresh flat-leaf parsley, chopped

1 tbsp freshly squeezed lemon juice

2 tsp smoked paprika

pinch of cayenne pepper (optional)

Himalayan pink rock salt and freshly ground black pepper

3 red peppers, sliced in half and deseeded

classic tomato salsa (page 149), to serve

A naturally gluten-free grain, millet is also alkalising and easy to digest. Our blood and body cells naturally prefer a more alkaline environment to function at their strongest and healthiest. Most plant foods are alkalising, while animal products leave an acidic residue when they're metabolised. If you're a meat-eater, then these roast millet stuffed peppers are a great plant-based dish to help balance out your system. I added the walnuts and kale to add density, protein and beauty minerals to the dish, which I like to have with a big green salad for the added benefits of raw greens.

1 To cook the millet, rinse it well in a sieve. Place the water in a saucepan, add in the millet and bring to the boil over a medium-high heat. Reduce the heat, cover partly with a lid and simmer for 10–15 minutes, until the millet seeds have swollen and the water has almost boiled off. Remove from the heat and allow the remaining bit of water to be absorbed.

2 While the millet is cooking, preheat the oven to 220°C. Lightly grease a baking tray with coconut oil.

3 Heat the coconut oil in a saucepan over a medium heat. Sauté the onion and garlic for 5 minutes, then add the chopped carrots and cook for 6–8 minutes more, until the onion is lightly browned.

4 Place the cooked millet in a mixing bowl along with the sautéed onions, carrots and garlic. Add the chopped kale, walnuts, parsley, lemon juice, smoked paprika, a pinch of cayenne and some salt and pepper. Mix together well.

5 Place the halved peppers on the greased baking tray and fill each half with the millet stuffing. Bake for 20–25 minutes, until the top begins to turn brown.

6 Serve hot with some classic tomato salsa on the side and a green salad.

FIBRE-RICH BAKED FALAFELS

Serves 2

coconut oil, for greasing

330g cooked chickpeas
(see page 22 for cooking
instructions)

1 small red onion, diced

2 cloves of garlic, peeled

2 tbsp chopped fresh
coriander

2 tbsp chopped fresh parsley

1 tsp ground coriander

1 tsp ground cumin

1 tsp chilli powder

$1/2$ tsp ground turmeric

pinch of cayenne pepper

Himalayan pink rock salt and
freshly ground black pepper

90g chickpea flour (any other
gluten-free flour works too)

Moroccan-spiced carrot
guacamole (page 154),
to serve (optional)

citrus tahini dressing (page
143), to serve (optional)

Falafel is a hugely popular Middle Eastern dish made with chickpeas and usually fried. Chickpeas are naturally low in fat and high in fibre, and they're just as delicious and far kinder to your waistline when baked without all that excess oil. They make a great snack dipped in Moroccan-spiced carrot guacamole or served on top of salads with a drizzle of citrus tahini dressing.w

1   Preheat the oven to 190°C. Lightly grease a baking tray with coconut oil.
2   Blend the cooked chickpeas, onion and garlic in a food processor or blender until it forms a thick paste. Transfer to a bowl and add in the fresh herbs, spices and seasoning. Mix together well. Add the flour slowly, stirring it in continuously until the mixture thickens and holds together.
3   Use a tablespoon to scoop the mixture and roll it into balls in your hands. Lay them out on the greased tray and bake for 20–25 minutes, making sure to turn them over after 10–12 minutes. They should be golden brown.
4   Serve with Moroccan-spiced carrot guacamole as a dip or drizzled with citrus tahini dressing.

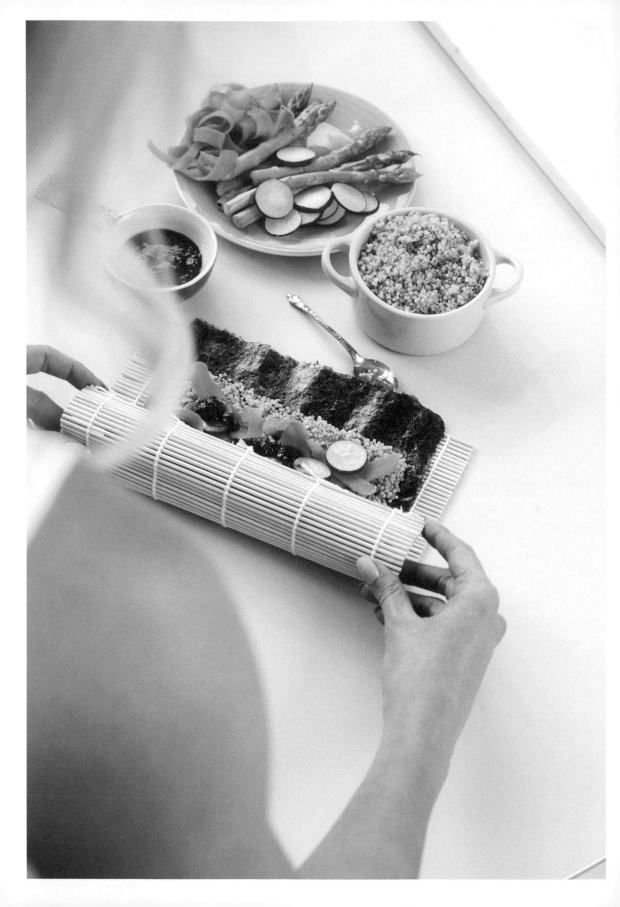

METABOLISM-BOOSTING QUINOA SUSHI WITH A GINGER MISO SAUCE

Serves 2

170g quinoa

500ml water

8 tbsp rice vinegar

4–5 drops of liquid stevia

pinch of Himalayan pink rock salt

4 sheets of nori seaweed

6 raw asparagus spears, chopped

2 medium carrots, peeled into ribbons and grated

2 radishes, thinly sliced

1 ripe avocado, peeled, pitted and sliced

1/2 cucumber, peeled and finely sliced

10g fresh coriander, chopped

FOR THE GINGER MISO SAUCE:

1 tsp sesame seeds, toasted

juice of 1 lime

4 drops of liquid stevia

2 tbsp organic miso paste

1 tsp finely grated fresh ginger

1 tsp low-sodium tamari sauce

I eat sea vegetables at least four times a week and I often advise my clients, friends and family to do the same. Not only are they full of beauty-enhancing fibre, vitamins and minerals, they're also a rich source of iodine. This mineral is essential to our thyroid's ability to manufacture thyroxine, which controls the metabolism of every cell in our body. I use a bamboo mat for rolling the sushi, which are widely available in good supermarkets or Asian food stores.

1 Rinse the quinoa well in a sieve and place it in a saucepan with the water. Bring it to the boil, then lower the heat, cover partly with a lid and simmer for 10–15 minutes, until the quinoa seeds have opened up and most of the water has evaporated. Remove from the heat and add the rice vinegar, stevia and a pinch of salt. Mix well and cover to allow the quinoa to absorb the flavours.

2 To put together the sushi rolls, place a bamboo mat on a flat countertop. Place a sheet of nori on the mat, then spread a layer of quinoa along the side closest to you, leaving a little space clear at the edge.

3 Place some asparagus, carrot ribbons, radishes, sliced avocado, sliced cucumber and coriander in a neat row in the middle of the nori. Start rolling with the side closest to you, using the mat to support it as you gently roll the quinoa over the vegetable filling. Ensure it's tightly rolled.

4 Dip your fingers in a little water and run them along the edge of the nori roll to seal the edges together. Use a sharp serrated knife to carefully cut the sushi into six slices.

5 To make the ginger miso sauce, toast the sesame seeds in a small, dry pan over a medium heat just until they start to turn golden. Take care not to burn them. Place in a small bowl and mix with the remaining sauce ingredients. Either drizzle it over the sushi before you roll it up or use it as a dip.

SKIN-GLOW SWEET POTATO COTTAGE PIE

Serves 6

1 tbsp organic virgin coconut oil, plus extra for greasing

1 medium red onion, diced

2 cloves of garlic, unpeeled and left whole

300g red lentils

1 litre low-sodium vegetable stock

1 tsp dried thyme

1 tsp ground cumin

Himalayan pink rock salt and freshly ground black pepper

220g frozen peas

3 medium carrots, peeled and cut into bite-sized pieces

3 tbsp chopped fresh parsley, to garnish

FOR THE SWEET POTATO MASH:

3 cloves of garlic, unpeeled

1.2kg sweet potatoes (about 8 medium or large sweet potatoes)

juice of 1 large orange

1 tbsp chopped fresh ginger

2 tsp ground turmeric

Thanks to their fibre, protein, antioxidants and iron, lentils make a satisfying and 'meaty' alternative to ground beef in vegan-friendly dishes like cottage pies and lasagnes. I've added that versatile old favourite, sweet potato, as the topping. It's a healthier alternative to white potatoes, but the triple whammy of orange, ginger and turmeric as well as the roast garlic makes it a superstar for glowing skin and a strong immune system. This recipe serves six, as I find it easier to make a larger portion and eat the leftovers the following day, plus it freezes well too.

1   Preheat the oven to 200°C. Lightly grease a 28cm x 18cm baking dish with coconut oil.
2   To make the mash, roast the unpeeled whole garlic cloves for 15–20 minutes in a small tray, until they are lightly browned and soft. Remove from the oven but leave it on.
3   Scrub the sweet potatoes and slice into halves and then quarters. Place in a large pot and fill with water just until the potatoes are covered. Bring to a gentle boil, then reduce the heat to a simmer, cover and allow the sweet potatoes to cook for about 15 minutes, until they can be easily sliced. When cooked through, drain well to remove any lingering water and place in a large mixing bowl. Use a potato masher or fork to mash well, then mix in the orange juice, ginger and turmeric. Peel the skins off the roast garlic cloves and mash the garlic into the sweet potatoes. Place the bowl to one side.
4   Set a large saucepan over a medium heat and melt the coconut oil. Sauté the onion and garlic for 4–5 minutes, until lightly browned. Pour in the lentils, vegetable stock, thyme, cumin and some salt and pepper and mix well. Bring to the boil, then cover partly with a lid, reduce the heat and simmer for 30 minutes.

5   After 30 minutes of cooking, pour in the frozen peas and chopped carrots. Stir well, cover the saucepan and continue to simmer for an additional 10 minutes, until the lentils and carrots are soft.

6   For a thicker lentil mixture, add in 2 tablespoons of the mashed sweet potatoes and mix well. Pour the lentils into the greased baking dish and spoon the mashed potatoes on top, ensuring it's smooth and even. Sprinkle a little more salt and pepper on top if desired.

7   Cook in the oven for 15 minutes, until the top turns golden brown. Remove from the oven and let it cool briefly before serving. Garnish with the chopped parsley and serve with a green salad.

PROTEIN-PACKED QUINOA, LENTIL AND APPLE GRIDDLE CAKES

Serves 5–6

200g Puy lentils

170g quinoa

150ml water

1 clove of garlic, minced

1 tbsp raw virgin coconut oil, plus extra for cooking

1 tbsp chopped fresh coriander

1 tbsp freshly squeezed lemon juice

1 tbsp raw apple cider vinegar

2 tsp ground cumin

1 1/2 tsp coriander seeds, crushed

1 tsp minced fresh ginger

1 tsp ground turmeric

1 tsp chilli flakes

3/4 tsp gluten-free baking powder

Himalayan pink rock salt and freshly ground black pepper

1/2 medium apple, grated

3 tbsp finely diced red onion

raw greens, to serve

citrus tahini dressing (page 141), to serve

Whether you're a meat-eater or plant-muncher, lentils are a brilliant addition to any diet. They're not only a source of complete protein and crammed with fibre and antioxidants, they're also a naturally low-calorie and low-fat food with none of the saturated fat and cholesterol found in meat, poultry and other animal products. Quinoa is a similarly valuable plant-based source of all eight amino acids. The warming spices and apple add a gentle sweetness and fragrance to the griddle cakes, which I love to eat with a big green salad and a drizzle of my citrus tahini dressing..

1 First soak the lentils for 8 hours or overnight. Place them in a bowl and cover with cold water, leaving 2.5cm of room at the top of the bowl to allow for the lentils to expand and absorb the liquid. After soaking, drain the lentils and rinse them.

2 Rinse the quinoa well in a sieve to prepare it for cooking. Place the lentils and quinoa into a blender or food processor along with the water, garlic, coconut oil, fresh coriander, lemon juice, apple cider vinegar, cumin, crushed coriander seeds, ginger, turmeric, chilli flakes, baking powder and some salt and pepper. Blend until the mixture is totally smooth. Pour into a large mixing bowl and stir in the grated apple and finely diced red onion.

3 Lightly grease a frying pan with coconut oil and melt it over a medium heat. Use a ladle to drop some mixture onto the hot pan. Cook for 2 minutes before flipping it over and cooking the other side for 2 minutes more, until golden brown on both sides. I like to make smaller, thicker griddle cakes.

4 Continue until the batter is used up, transferring each griddle cake to a plate lined with a few sheets of kitchen paper to absorb any extra oil.

5 Serve with raw greens and a drizzle of citrus tahini dressing to enhance the flavour of the spices.

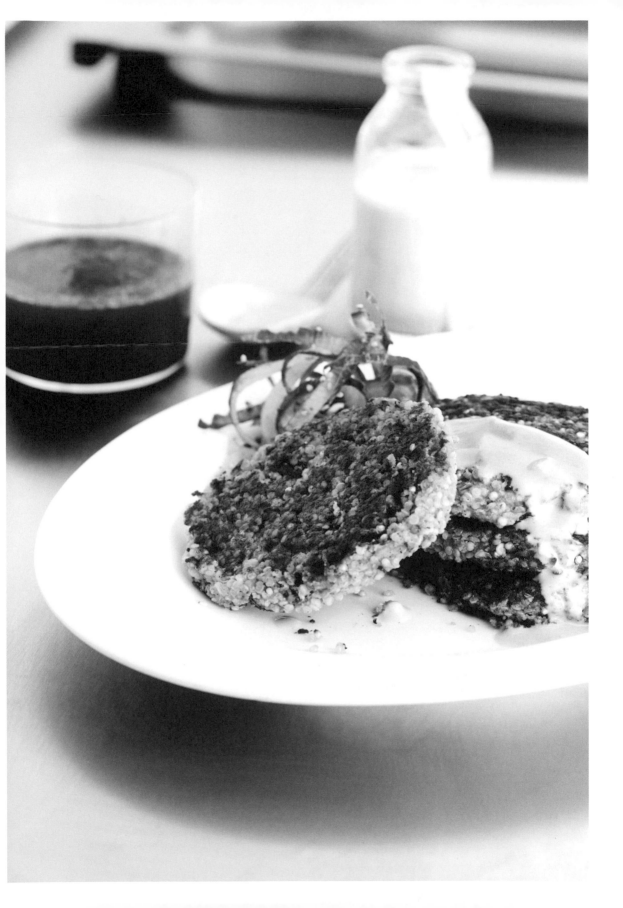

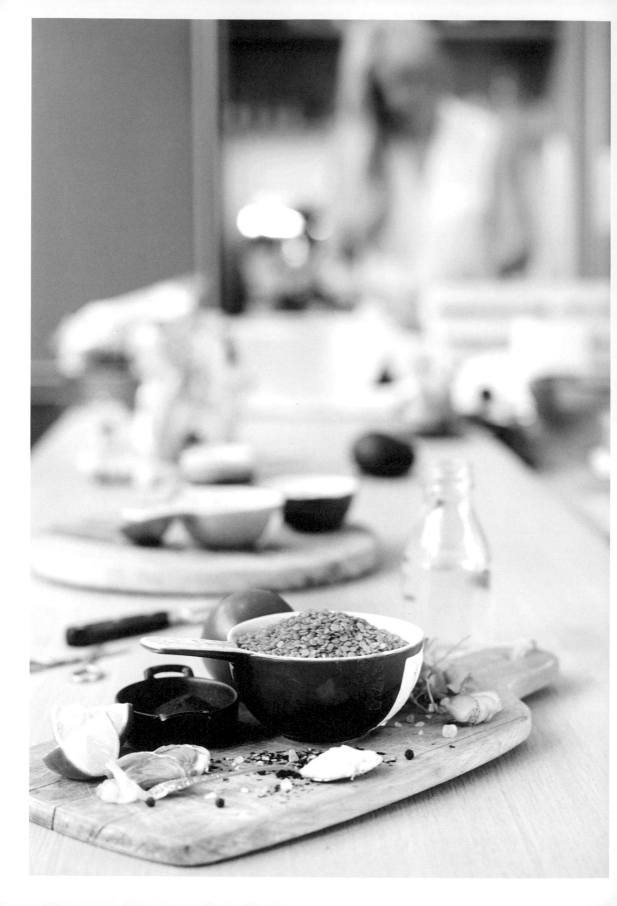

COCONUT AND CORIANDER RED LENTIL DAHL

Serves 5–6

400g red lentils

1/2 tbsp organic virgin coconut oil

2 small red onions or 1 large, diced

3 cloves of garlic, minced

1 tbsp finely chopped fresh ginger

2 ripe, medium tomatoes, chopped

2 tsp curry powder

1 tsp ground turmeric

1 tsp smoked paprika

1/2 tsp chilli flakes

700ml water

400ml low-fat coconut milk

Himalayan pink rock salt and freshly ground black pepper

freshly squeezed lime juice, to serve

20g toasted coconut flakes, to garnish

4 tbsp chopped fresh coriander, to garnish

This is one of my favourite healthy comfort meals, as it's so nourishing and simple to make. Protein- and fibre-filled lentils, liver-detoxifying coriander, metabolism-boosting chilli, lycopene-rich cooked tomatoes and fragrant spices are all fused together in a big bowl of warming goodness.

1   First soak the lentils for 8 hours or overnight. Place them in a bowl and cover with cold water, leaving 2.5cm of room at the top of the bowl to allow for the lentils to expand and absorb the liquid. After soaking, drain the lentils and rinse them well.

2   Heat the coconut oil in a saucepan over a medium heat. Cook the onions, garlic and ginger, stirring frequently, for 5 minutes, until lightly browned. Add in the chopped tomatoes, spices, water, coconut milk and drained lentils and season with salt and pepper. Bring to the boil over a medium-high heat, then reduce the heat and allow it to simmer gently for 35–40 minutes, until it thickens up and the lentils have softened.

3   Remove from the heat and add a squeeze of fresh lime juice. Garnish with the toasted coconut flakes and a sprinkle of fresh coriander. Serve with a green salad and quinoa or brown rice.

BLOOD-CLEANSING BEETROOT CRISPS WITH LEMON AND PARSLEY HUMMUS

Serves 2

2 large beetroot, peeled and cut into crisps or rectangular chips

1 tbsp raw virgin coconut oil, melted

$^1/_2$ tsp smoked paprika

pinch of Himalayan pink rock salt

lemon and parsley hummus (page 145)

Beetroot is an incredible vegetable for building your blood and cleansing it of the toxins that can cause disease. I aim to eat at least one or two servings of beetroot every week in smoothies, salads or simply roasted, as in this recipe. They have a sweet, earthy flavour that pairs well with my lemon and parsley hummus. I also like to cut the beetroot into crisps or chips and dip them into a small bowl of the hummus for a snack or light meal.

1   Preheat the oven to 190°C.
2   Place the beetroot crisps or chips on a baking tray and toss them in the melted coconut oil, smoked paprika and a pinch of salt.
3   Roast in the oven for 25–30 minutes, turning them over after 15 minutes. Remove from the oven when they are beginning to turn brown.
4   Serve warm with a bowl of lemon and parsley hummus for dipping them into.

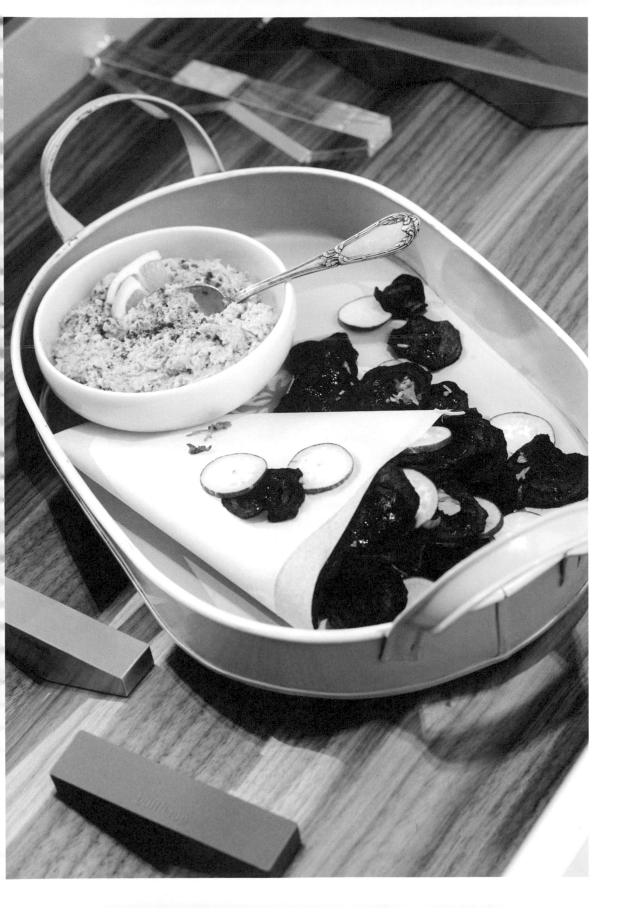

KIDNEY BEAN AND QUINOA BURGERS

Makes 4 burgers

coconut oil, for greasing

1 tbsp ground flaxseed

250ml + 2 tbsp cold water

85g quinoa

425g cooked kidney beans (see page 22 for cooking instructions)

90g buckwheat flour

65g fresh or frozen peas

1 small red onion, finely diced

1/2 red pepper, seeds removed and finely diced

1 clove of garlic, crushed

juice of 1 lemon

1 tbsp dried oregano

1 tsp smoked paprika

Himalayan pink rock salt and freshly ground black pepper

zesty guacamole (page 153), to serve

sliced tomatoes, to serve

large lettuce leaves, to serve

A hearty veggie burger is an ideal option for bigger appetites and even carnivores looking for a satisfying plant-based meal with a meaty texture. These low-fat kidney bean and quinoa burgers are really filling and are an excellent source of fibre, slow-release carbohydrates and a complete source of plant protein. The burgers are also a cheap and easy way to use up leftover quinoa, veggies and that bag of kidney beans sitting in the back of your cupboard.

1 Preheat the oven to 190°C. Lightly grease a baking tray with coconut oil.

2 Prepare the flax 'egg' by placing the ground flaxseed in a small bowl and mixing with 2 tablespoons of water. Place in the fridge for 10 minutes to set.

3 Rinse the quinoa well in a sieve and place it in a saucepan with the 250ml of water. Bring it to the boil, then lower the heat, cover the pan and simmer for 10–15 minutes, until the quinoa seeds have opened up and most of the water has evaporated. Remove from the heat and allow it to sit for up to 10 minutes to absorb the rest of the water.

4 Mash the cooked kidney beans in a bowl, allowing some chunks to remain.

5 Transfer the cooked quinoa to a large bowl. Add the mashed beans, buckwheat flour, peas, red onion, red pepper, garlic, lemon juice, oregano, smoked paprika, the flax 'egg' and some salt and pepper and mix well until combined. Taste at this point to see if you would prefer more seasoning.

6 Divide the mixture into four sections with a knife. Roll each section into a ball and then flatten into a burger patty. Place the burgers on the greased baking tray.

7 Bake the burgers for 30 minutes, turning them over after 15 minutes.

8 Transfer to a serving plate and top the burgers with zesty guacamole and a slice of fresh tomato sprinkled with a little freshly ground black pepper. I like to wrap them in large lettuce leaves to serve.

QUINOA COLOUR DOME WITH SKIN-BRIGHTENING SMOKY SWEET PEPPER AND WALNUT DIP

Serves 2

170g quinoa

500ml water

1 medium sweet potato, unpeeled and cut into bite-sized cubes

1/2 tbsp organic virgin coconut oil, melted

2 tsp smoked paprika, plus an extra pinch to garnish

Himalayan pink rock salt and freshly ground black pepper

1 ripe avocado, pitted, peeled and cut into cubes

juice of 1 lime

pinch of dried chilli flakes

smoky sweet pepper and walnut dip (page 143), to serve

2 tbsp chopped fresh coriander, to garnish

This is a deceptively simple meal that incorporates all the protein-packed goodness of quinoa for a lean, toned body with the skin-smoothing, healing and brightening benefits of the avocado, sweet potato and the walnut and sweet pepper sauce. It's also one of my favourite dishes to serve when I want to impress my friends and family, due to its variety of colours and flavours.

1 Rinse the quinoa well in a sieve and place it in a saucepan with the water. Bring it to the boil, then cover partly with a lid, lower the heat and simmer for 10–15 minutes, until the quinoa seeds have opened up and most of the water has evaporated. Remove from the heat and allow it to sit, covered, for up to 10 minutes to absorb the rest of the water.

2 Preheat the oven to 210°C.

3 Arrange the sweet potato cubes on a baking tray and drizzle with the melted coconut oil. Sprinkle on the smoked paprika and seasoning and toss, ensuring each piece is coated with spices and oil. Bake in the oven for 30–35 minutes, until lightly browned and crispy.

4 Place the diced avocado in a small bowl with a squeeze of lime juice, a pinch of chilli flakes and some salt and pepper.

5 To serve, press the cooked quinoa firmly into a small dish or cereal bowl. Place a dinner plate across the top of the bowl and flip the whole thing over so that the quinoa comes out on the plate in the shape of a dome.

6 Arrange the baked sweet potato cubes on top of the quinoa, then add the avocado on top of the sweet potato. Drizzle the walnut and sweet pepper sauce on top of everything and garnish with a sprinkle of smoked paprika and the chopped coriander.

DESSERTS AND SWEET TREATS

We all deserve a treat from time to time, and the *Eat Yourself Beautiful* programme encourages an indulgent sweet treat once a week. Plus they taste so much better when you look forward to them for a few days and let the anticipation build. As with all my recipes, my desserts and sweet snacks are free from the dairy, gluten, refined sugar, trans fats, chemicals and preservatives found in many commercial recipes. I've chosen each and every ingredient for their health and beauty benefits, as most of them are rich in nutrients and antioxidants. However, they are also rich in calories, so they must be treated as a special indulgence if you want to look and feel your very best.

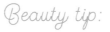

Beauty tip:

ALWAYS **SOAK NUTS AND SEEDS** IN A
BOWL OF FRESH WATER FOR A FEW HOURS
OR OVERNIGHT AND RINSE WELL BEFORE
EATING TO REMOVE THE INHIBITOR ENZYMES
ON THEIR SKIN, WHICH NATURALLY PROTECT
THE NUT FROM GERMINATING UNTIL THE
CONDITIONS ARE OPTIMAL. THIS REALLY
HELPS TO IMPROVE THEIR DIGESTION AND
MAKES THEM MORE ALKALISING SO THAT
YOU CAN BENEFIT MORE FROM THEIR ARRAY
OF NUTRIENTS. STORE THEM IN THE FRIDGE
FOR MAXIMUM FRESHNESS.

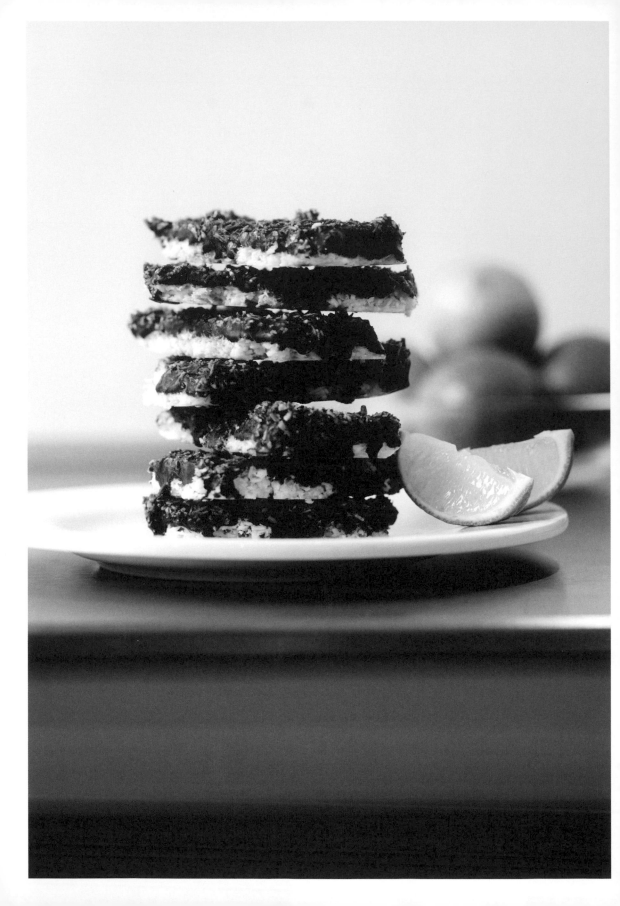

TASTE OF THE TROPICS COCONUT BARS

Makes 8 bars

FOR THE BARS:

200g unsweetened desiccated coconut

100g coconut oil

50g organic maple syrup, coconut nectar or local raw honey (if you're not vegan)

FOR THE DARK CHOCOLATE TOPPING:

220g cacao butter

80g raw cacao powder

80g pure maple syrup

5 drops of liquid stevia (optional)

I spend so much time dreaming of the colours, warmth and tastes of tropical lands that these bars are pretty much the perfect treat to whip up on a cold rainy day at home. I just lie back, close my eyes and pretend I'm swinging gently in a hammock below the palm trees. Cacao butter is available in good health food shops. It's the edible fat left behind when the cacao solids are removed. Coconut and raw cacao are such skin superfoods that these special occasion treat bars do as much good for your complexion as they do for your taste buds.

1   To make the bars, line a 24cm x 24cm square tin with grease-proof paper. Place the desiccated coconut, coconut oil and maple syrup in a bowl and use a spoon or fork to mash them together until well mixed. Press into the lined tin and place in the freezer for 20–30 minutes, until solid.

2   Meanwhile, to make the topping, melt the cacao butter in a small saucepan over a medium heat. Add the cacao powder and whisk together until there are no lumps. Add the maple syrup and whisk again. Add the liquid stevia if a sweeter taste is desired.

3   Remove the tin from the freezer and cut the mixture into eight bars. Dip each bar into the dark chocolate mixture. Lay the bars on a piece of greaseproof paper and place in the fridge for 30 minutes to allow the chocolate to set.

4   Keep refrigerated in an airtight container for up to four days and serve chilled.

SUMMER BERRY ICE CREAM WITH CHOCOLATE MAPLE SAUCE

Serves 2

FOR THE ICE CREAM:

125g frozen mixed berries

2 bananas, peeled, chopped and frozen

2 Medjool dates, pitted

4 tbsp cashew nuts

2 tsp vanilla extract

250ml chilled coconut water

2 tbsp goji berries, to serve

FOR THE CHOCOLATE MAPLE SAUCE:

2 tbsp melted organic virgin coconut oil

2 tbsp raw cacao powder

2 tbsp tahini

2 tbsp pure organic maple syrup

Classic ice cream and chocolate sauce served with a fruity twist, perfect for summer garden parties. The chocolate sauce freezes onto the ice cream for a delightfully decadent crunch.

1. To make the ice cream, put the berries, frozen bananas, dates, cashews and vanilla extract in a blender and combine well. Add the coconut water slowly to achieve a smooth and creamy consistency. Depending on your blender, you might not need all of the coconut water. Transfer the ice cream to a bowl and keep it in the freezer while you prepare the chocolate maple sauce.
2. Melt the coconut oil in a small saucepan over a medium heat. Remove from the heat and stir in the cacao powder, tahini and maple syrup until it becomes a smooth chocolate sauce.
3. Divide the ice cream between two bowls. Drizzle the sauce over it, top with goji berries and serve immediately.

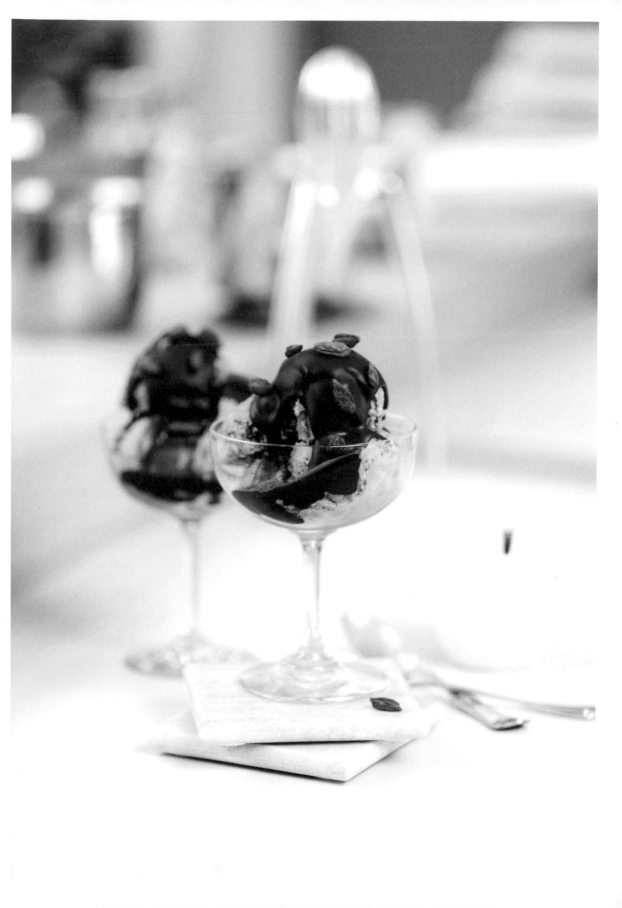

NUTTY CINNAMON RAISIN COOKIES

Makes 12 cookies

60g skinned hazelnuts

90g organic raisins

30g gluten-free rolled oats

20g unsweetened desiccated coconut

3 tbsp pitted and chopped dates

2 tbsp ground flaxseed

1 tbsp organic maple syrup or coconut palm nectar

1 tbsp melted coconut oil, plus extra for greasing

2 tsp ground cinnamon

1 tsp vanilla extract

I often make these crunchy spiced cookies around Christmas-time for family and friends because they have such a warm, cosy, homely taste and are always a people-pleaser. Both delicious and nourishing for skin and hair, it can be difficult to stop at just one!

1   Preheat the oven to 190°C. Lightly grease two baking trays with coconut oil.
2   Spread out the hazelnuts on a baking tray and place in the oven for 5–10 minutes, until lightly toasted. Set aside to cool.
3   Place all the ingredients in a blender or food processor and blend until it forms a sticky dough.
4   Roll into individual balls using 2 tablespoons of the cookie dough. Place each ball on the greased baking trays and press down gently to form a disc. Alternatively, you could roll out the dough and use a cookie cutter to form shapes.
5   Bake in the oven for 15–20 minutes, until the cookies are golden brown. Remove from the oven and let the cookies cool on the tray for a few minutes before carefully transferring them to a wire cooling rack.
6   Store in an airtight container for up to three days.

MAPLE, WALNUT AND CINNAMON ICE CREAM

Serves 2

4 bananas, peeled, chopped into chunks and frozen

3–4 tbsp unsweetened almond milk

1 tsp ground cinnamon

1 tsp vanilla seeds or pure vanilla extract

2 tbsp chopped walnuts, to serve

1–2 tbsp pure organic maple syrup, to serve

pinch of cinnamon, to serve

This recipe is a proper people-pleaser and the perfect dessert when friends pop over for a casual supper. It's ridiculously easy to whizz up and the frozen bananas blend together to create the exact same texture as regular ice cream. It's hard to beat the flavour of real vanilla seeds, but a pure vanilla extract works well too. I've added raw walnuts for their skin-boosting qualities and cinnamon for its blood sugar-balancing benefits. The maple syrup is totally optional, but a little drizzle tastes so good. A little raw honey or coconut nectar are other recommended sweetener options.

1 Place the frozen banana chunks, almond milk, cinnamon and vanilla in a blender and combine until the mixture is smooth, creamy and resembles ice cream in texture.

2 Serve immediately in bowls topped with chopped walnuts, a drizzle of maple syrup and a sprinkle of cinnamon. Any leftovers can be stored in a covered container in the freezer for up to three months.

RAW CHOCOLATE AND SALTED CARAMEL SLICE

Makes 6–8 squares

FOR THE BASE:

150g dates, pitted and chopped

110g unsalted almonds

1 tsp ground cinnamon

1 tsp organic virgin coconut oil

FOR THE SALTED CARAMEL LAYER:

130g cashews

150g dates, pitted and chopped

150g pure organic maple syrup

110g organic virgin coconut oil

80ml water

1¹/₂ tbsp tahini

1 tsp pure vanilla extract

pinch of Himalayan pink rock salt

FOR THE CHOCOLATE TOPPING:

75g pure organic maple syrup

55g organic virgin coconut oil

30g raw cacao powder

sliced fresh strawberries, to serve

As a child, my absolute favourite sweet treat was a chocolate caramel slice, which I might get on a Sunday after lunch if I was very lucky. I loved the different layers of rich chocolate, gooey melting caramel and the biscuity base. These chocolate salted caramel slices are so similar to the version I used to eat, but using only whole, plant-based ingredients. Raw, vegan and free from refined sugar, dairy, gluten and trans fats, they're a special treat.

1   Lightly grease a 24cm x 24cm square tin with coconut oil or line with greaseproof paper.

2   For the base, soak the chopped dates in a small bowl of warm water for 15–20 minutes to soften. Drain the dates and place them in a blender or food processor with the almonds, cinnamon and coconut oil and blend until the mixture becomes sticky crumbs. Pour into the prepared tin. Ensure it's even and press down firmly. Place it in the freezer to set.

3   Meanwhile, soak the cashew nuts for 1 hour in a small bowl of water. Soak the chopped dates in a separate small bowl of lukewarm water for 15–20 minutes to soften them. Drain the nuts and the dates.

4   Place the soaked cashews and dates into a blender or food processor with the maple syrup, coconut oil, water, tahini, vanilla extract and a pinch of salt. Blend until smooth. Use a little extra water if necessary to help it combine. Pour the caramel layer onto the base layer, spread it out evenly and return to the freezer to set.

5   Once the caramel layer has set, make the chocolate topping. Combine the maple syrup, coconut oil and cacao powder in a small saucepan set on a low heat until it looks like chocolate sauce. Pour the chocolate sauce over the caramel layer and ensure it's even. Place it back in the freezer for another 1–2 hours, until completely set.

6   Slice into six or eight squares with a sharp knife. Serve with a sliced fresh strawberry on top. Store in a covered container in the fridge for up to four days.

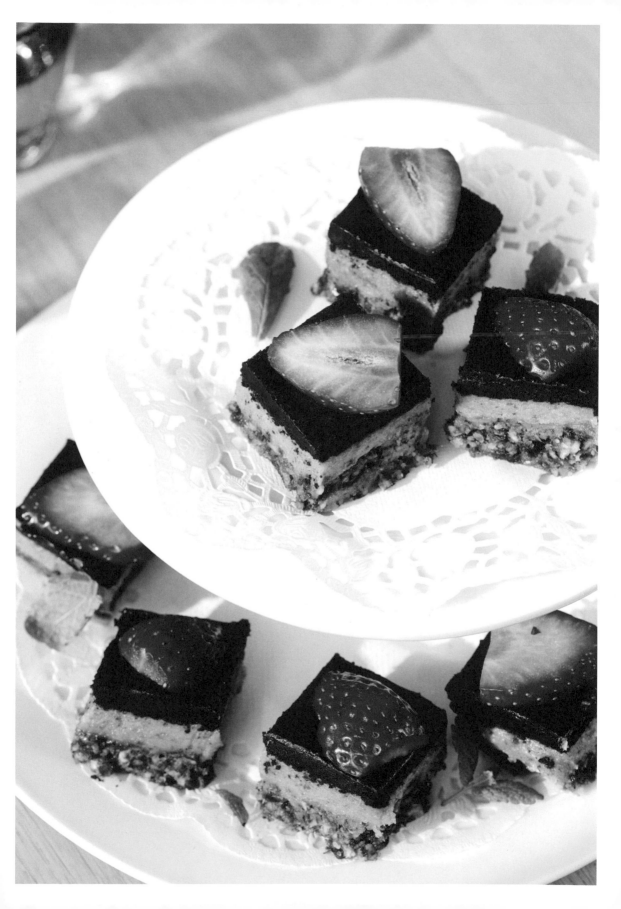

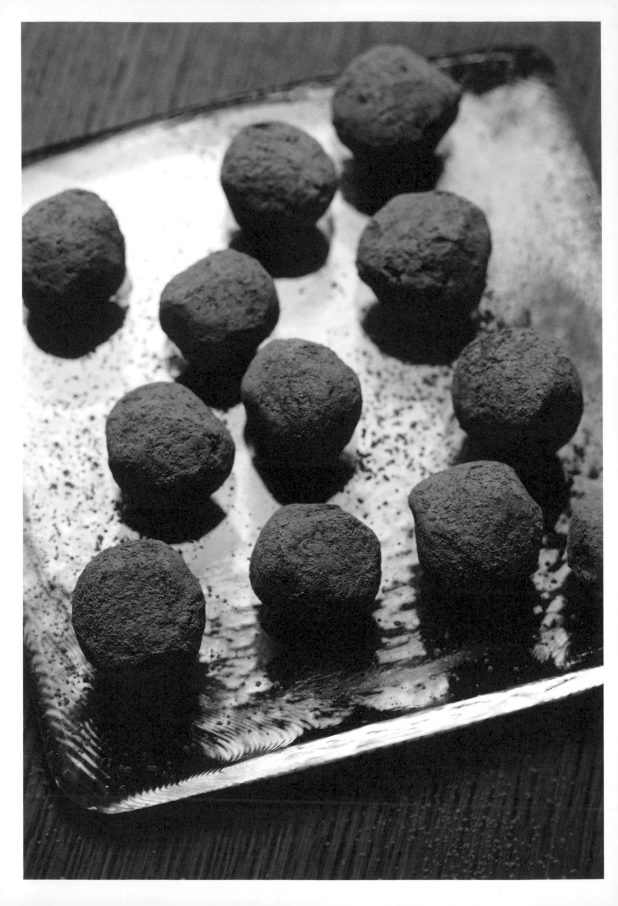

CACAO HAZELNUT BLISS BALLS

Makes 8–10 balls

175g skinned hazelnuts

75g dates, pitted and chopped

30g raw cacao powder, plus extra for rolling

2–3 tbsp pure organic maple syrup or coconut nectar (optional)

1 tbsp tahini

Simple, straightforward, but oh so delicious! These bliss balls hit the spot when something a little creamy and chocolaty is required. But with ingredients that include antioxidant-rich raw cacao powder and calcium-filled tahini, you can enjoy these totally guilt free.

1 Preheat the oven to 190°C.
2 Spread out the hazelnuts on a baking tray and place in the oven for 5–10 minutes, until lightly toasted. Set side to cool.
3 Soak the chopped dates in a small bowl of warm water for 15–20 minutes to soften them. Drain well.
4 Place the toasted hazelnuts, soaked dates, cacao powder, the sweetener (if using) and the tahini in a blender or food processor. Blend until the mixture is well combined.
5 Put a little cacao powder in a shallow bowl. Roll the mixture into eight to ten individual balls and then roll the balls in cacao powder until fully covered.
6 Store in an airtight container in the fridge until ready to serve. These will keep for up to four days.

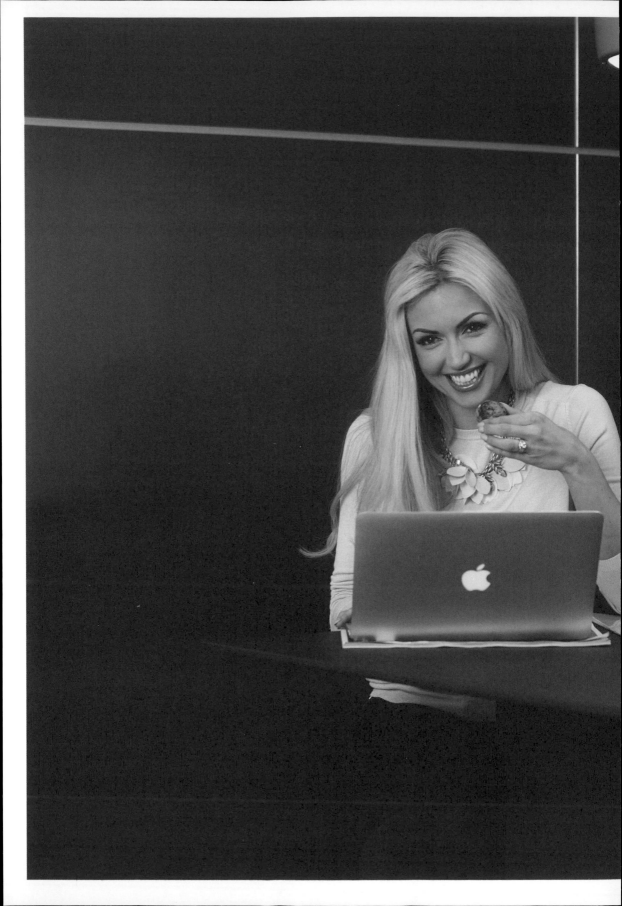

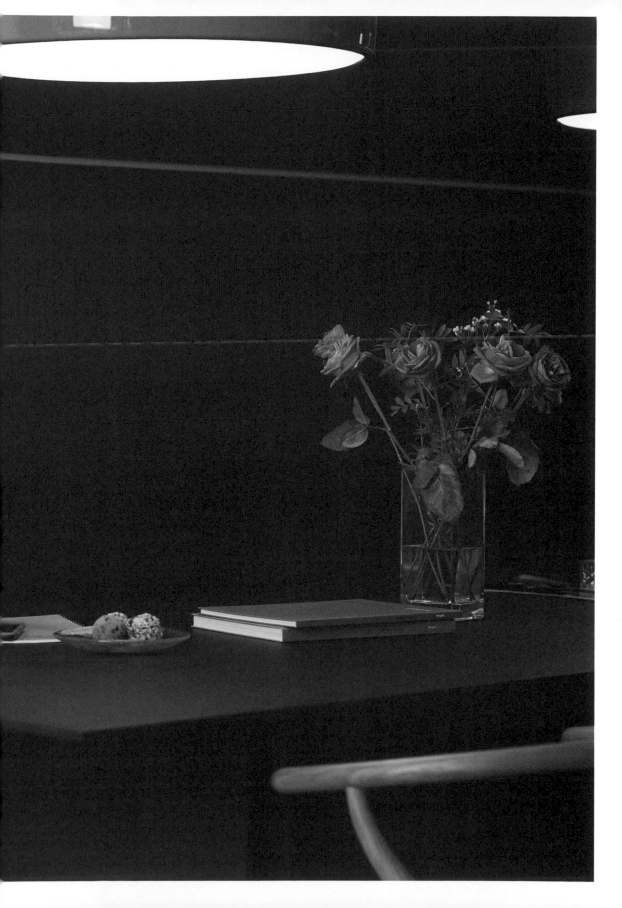

RAW CARROT CAKE WITH CITRUS CASHEW FROSTING

Serves 6

FOR THE CARROT CAKE:

235g gluten-free oats

3 large carrots, peeled and cut into chunks

300g pitted dates, chopped

60g raw walnuts, chopped

1 tsp ground cinnamon

$\frac{1}{2}$ tsp ground nutmeg

FOR THE CITRUS CASHEW FROSTING:

200g raw cashew nuts

juice of 1 lemon

2 tbsp melted coconut oil

2 tbsp organic maple syrup

1 tsp vanilla extract

about 50ml cold water

Growing up, carrot cake was one of my most-loved treats, and at least the carrots convinced me it was a little healthier. When I moved to a plant-based diet, carrot cake was one of the harder desserts to give up. But as with most confections, there is a more nutritious alternative to the waistline-sabotaging carrot cake that we all know. This version uses cashews to create an amazingly smooth and creamy icing with a lemony twist, while fibre-rich dates, walnuts, spices and oats are combined to form the carrot cake. It's the perfect dessert to whip up for special occasions to impress guests and it doesn't even need to be baked.

1   First make the frosting. Soak the cashews in a small bowl of cold water for 4 hours, then drain well. Combine all the frosting ingredients in a blender and add water as needed to create a smooth, creamy icing (I usually use about 50ml of cold water). When blended, transfer the icing to a bowl and put it in the fridge to set.

2   Cake next! Place the oats in your food processor or blender and blend until they become a flour. Pour out into a bowl.

3   Put the carrots, dates, walnuts and spices into the food processor or blender and blend until they begin to stick together and form a dough. Gradually add in the oat flour and blend until it's all well mixed. Remove and press firmly and evenly into a 24cm x 24cm silicone tray or a springform tin.

4   Ice the carrot cake with the cashew frosting and place into the freezer for 2 hours to set.

5   If you want to decorate your cake, I like to sprinkle mine with fresh blueberries and drizzle a little maple syrup across the top. Cut into slices and serve.

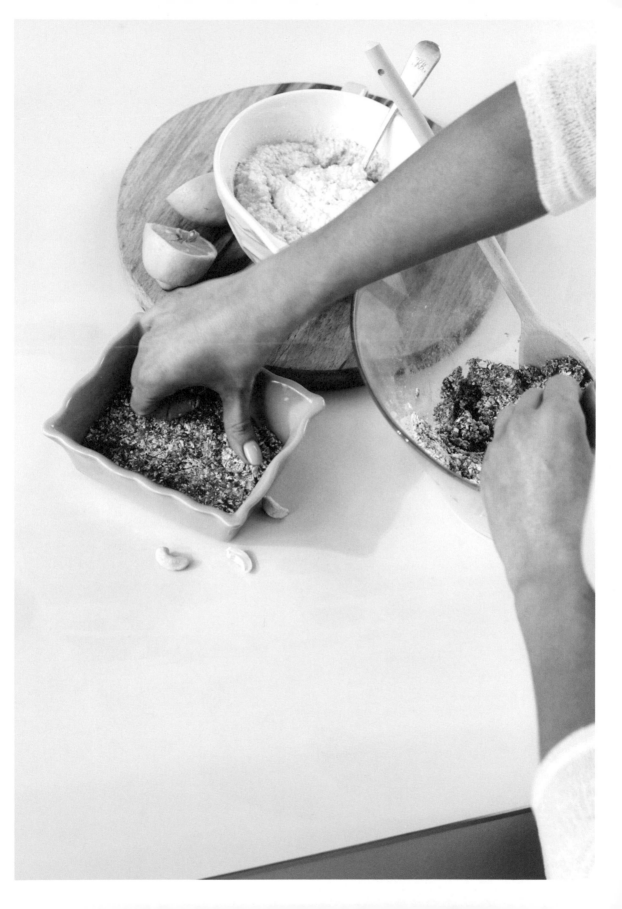

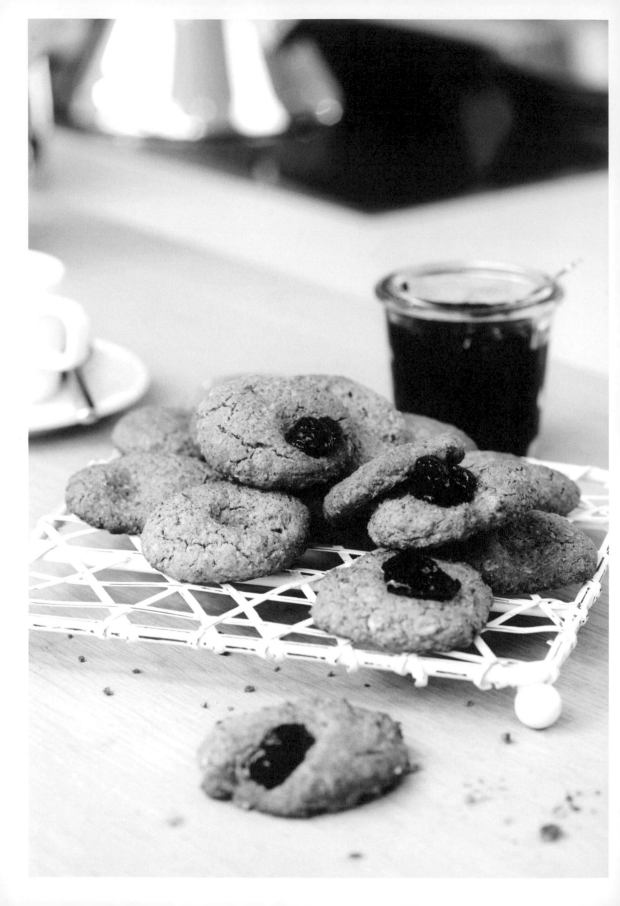

MINI ALMOND THUMB-PRINT COOKIES WITH BLUEBERRY CHIA JAM

Makes 10–12 cookies

FOR THE MINI ALMOND THUMBPRINT COOKIES:

coconut oil, for greasing

250g cooked chickpeas (see page 22 for cooking instructions)

125g raw unsalted almond butter

3 tbsp pure organic maple syrup or coconut nectar

2 tsp pure vanilla extract

1 tsp gluten-free baking powder

20g gluten-free rolled oats

FOR THE BLUEBERRY CHIA JAM:

1 tbsp pure maple syrup

250g frozen blueberries

juice of ½ lemon

2 tbsp chia seeds

Kids will love making these fun treats as the centre of the cookies are shaped using their thumbs and then filled with a sweet but healthy blueberry jam. They also make a great snack to stabilise blood sugar levels and slowly release energy thanks to their high protein content. I use chickpeas instead of flour because they give a density to the mixture and absorb all of the flavours added to them. The almonds in the almond butter provide plenty of antioxidant vitamin E to protect your skin from damaging UV light.

1   To make the blueberry chia jam, heat the maple syrup in a saucepan over a medium heat until it begins to gently bubble. Add the frozen blueberries and lemon juice, stirring well, and simmer until the berries begin to break down and liquefy. Taste at this point and add a little more maple syrup if you prefer it sweeter, though I like it quite tart. Add the chia seeds and stir well for 30–60 seconds. Turn off the heat and continue to stir until the chia seeds begin to absorb the liquid from the blueberries and swell up. Pour the jam into a container or jar and set in the fridge for 1 hour.

2   Preheat the oven to 180°C. Lightly grease a baking tray with coconut oil.

3   Place the cooked chickpeas, almond butter, maple syrup, vanilla extract and baking powder in a blender and whizz until it forms a smooth, thick batter. Pour the batter into a mixing bowl and stir in the oats until well combined.

4   Using your hands, roll the dough into 10 to 12 individual balls about the size of a ping pong ball. Place on the greased tray and press down with your palm to slightly flatten them. Using your thumb, press an indentation into the centre of each cookie.

5   Bake for 20–25 minutes, until the cookies are firm to touch. Remove from the oven and transfer to a wire rack to cool.

6   Add a teaspoon of blueberry chia jam to the indent of each cookie. Keep stored in an airtight container for up to three days.

LOW-FAT CHOCOLATE FUDGE BROWNIES

Makes 12–14 brownies

15 Medjool dates, pitted

coconut oil, for greasing

600g sweet potatoes (about 2 medium potatoes), peeled and cut in half

85g raw organic cacao powder

80g ground almonds

50g chopped walnuts (optional)

270ml unsweetened almond milk

2 tbsp good-quality maple syrup

1 tsp pure vanilla extract

pinch of Himalayan pink rock salt

100g buckwheat flour

1 tsp gluten-free baking powder

Chocolate brownies are traditionally a rich, decadent dessert, totally delicious but sinful for the waistline. Brownies are usually made with rich fats, refined sugar, melted chocolate and an assortment of other guilt-inducing goodies. These brownies are a little different but are still tasty, gooey and mouth-watering. They're 100% vegan, low fat and completely free from dairy, gluten, refined sugar, eggs, soya and oils. In fact, their chocolate fudge texture owes itself to one surprise superstar ingredient: sweet potatoes! They add a great fluffiness while absorbing the flavours of the raw cacao powder and sweet dates. Plus they're high in fibre, rich in beta-carotene and extremely good for health and beauty. It's a win-win.

1   Soak the dates in a small bowl of warm water for 15–20 minutes to soften. Drain well.

2   Preheat the oven to 210°C. Lightly grease a 24cm x 24cm square baking tin with coconut oil.

3   Steam the halved sweet potatoes for about 10 minutes, until soft.

4   Place the steamed sweet potatoes into a blender with the soaked dates, cacao powder, ground almonds, walnuts (if using), almond milk, maple syrup, vanilla extract and a pinch of salt. Blend together until smooth and pour into a bowl. Fold in the flour and baking powder until the batter reaches a thick consistency and pour into the greased baking tin.

5   Bake for 20–25 minutes, until the top is crisp and a knife inserted into the centre of the brownies comes out clean and dry.

6   Remove from the oven and allow to cool for a few minutes before slicing the brownies into squares and transferring to a wire cooling rack. Store the brownies in an airtight container in the fridge for up to four days.

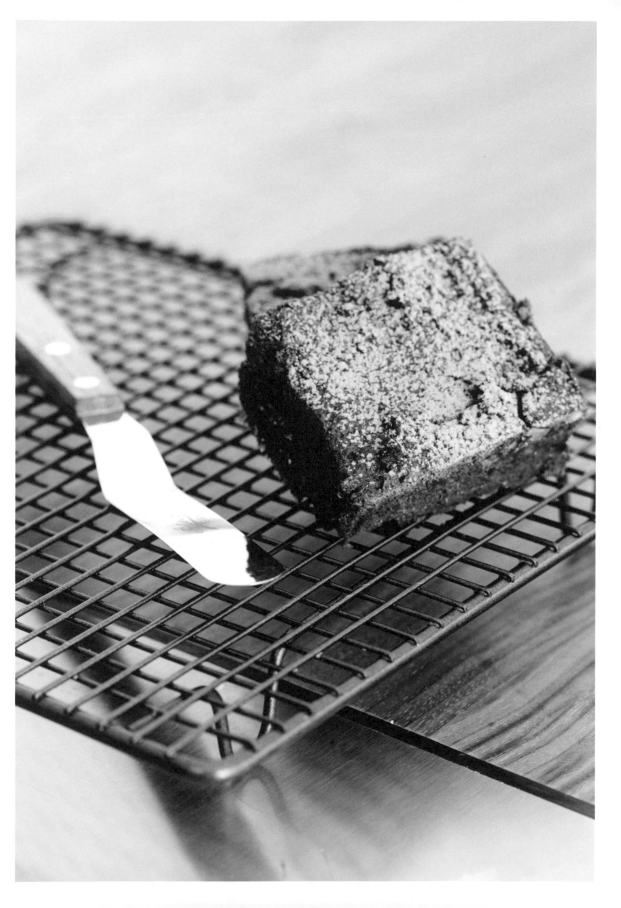

CRUNCHY CHOCOLATE AND MULBERRY ENERGY BITES

Makes 6–8 balls

200g pitted Medjool dates, chopped

150g dried white mulberries

2 tbsp raw cacao powder

1 tsp ground cinnamon

50g unsweetened desiccated coconut

These are great to grab on the go for a burst of energy and they contain plenty of tummy-flattening fibre. Mulberries make a tasty alternative to raisins and are packed with beautifying nutrients like potassium and vitamin C.

1 Soak the dates in a small bowl of warm water for 15–20 minutes to soften them. Drain well.

2 Place the drained dates, mulberries, cacao powder and cinnamon in a blender and combine together until they form a dough. Add a splash of water if necessary to help the ingredients blend.

3 Scoop up enough of the mixture to roll into a table tennis-size ball between the palms of your hands.

4 Place the coconut in a shallow bowl and roll each ball around in it to fully coat it.

5 Keep the balls in the fridge until ready to serve to allow the mulberries to get cold and crunchy. Stored in an airtight container in the fridge, these will keep for up to four days.

FROSTED SUPERFOOD GOJI BROWNIES

Makes 6–8 brownies

250g dates, pitted

75g gluten-free rolled oats

50g unsalted walnuts

6 tbsp raw organic cacao powder

2 tbsp unsweetened desiccated coconut

2 tbsp cold water

FOR THE BROWNIE ICING:

85g organic virgin coconut oil

3 tbsp raw organic cacao powder

3 tbsp pure organic maple syrup

1 tsp vanilla extract

3 heaped tbsp goji berries

These brownies are a great sweet treat as they're so easy to whip up, taste great and are free from nasties like refined sugar and trans fats. However, the ingredients may be nourishing but they're still rich, so please consider them an occasional indulgence! I have added coconut for its skin benefits and goji berries for their superfood properties, as they're a great source of vitamin C and health-protective antioxidants. They have also been used in Chinese medicine for centuries to treat age-related eye problems.

1   Soak the dates in a small bowl of warm water for 15–20 minutes to soften. Drain well.
2   Place the soaked dates in a blender or food processor with the oats, walnuts, cacao powder, coconut and cold water and blend until well mixed. Pour into a small tray (I use a square silicone tin). Place in the fridge to set.
3   Meanwhile, to make the icing, place all the ingredients except the goji berries in a blender or food processor and combine until smooth and creamy.
4   Pour the icing over the base and use a spatula to smooth it out. Sprinkle the goji berries across the top and place back into the fridge for 45 minutes to 1 hour, until completely set.
5   Cut the brownies into squares with a sharp knife and serve chilled. Store in an airtight container in the fridge for up to four days.

RICH RAW CHOCOLATE FLAPJACKS

Makes 6 flapjacks

FOR THE FLAPJACKS:

150g pitted dates, chopped

70g ground almonds

40g unsweetened desiccated coconut

2 heaped tbsp cacao powder

2 tbsp cacao nibs

1 tbsp maple syrup

1 tsp ground cinnamon

1 tsp vanilla extract

FOR THE CHOCOLATE TOPPING:

220g cacao butter

90g raw cacao powder

80g maple syrup

5 drops of liquid stevia (optional)

I absolutely love flapjacks and this is a great recipe to impress friends with when they pop over for a cup of tea. I used to make flapjacks as a little girl, but of course they were jammed with refined sugar and butter. This version keeps all of the rich flavour but uses nourishing raw superfood ingredients like coconut, almonds and cacao to create a truly scrumptious energy- and beauty-building sweet treat.

1. Soak the dates in a small bowl of warm water for 15–20 minutes to soften. Drain well.
2. Place the soaked dates, ground almonds, coconut, cacao powder, cacao nibs, maple syrup, cinnamon and vanilla extract in a food processor or blender. Blend until it's well mixed together. Pour into a square tin lined with greaseproof paper, spread out to your desired width and flatten evenly.
3. To make the chocolate topping, melt the cacao butter in a small saucepan over a medium heat. Add the cacao powder and whisk together until there are no lumps. Add the maple syrup and whisk again. Add the liquid stevia if a sweeter taste is desired.
4. Pour the chocolate sauce over the flapjacks. Place the tin in the fridge for 2–3 hours, until the flapjacks are firm. Remove from the tin and cut into six slices.

SEXY SKIN RAW CHOCOLATE TRUFFLES

Makes 10–12 truffles

300g Medjool dates, pitted

80g raw hulled hemp seeds

2 heaped tbsp raw organic cacao powder

2 tsp ground cinnamon

2 tsp vanilla extract

TO COAT:

2 tbsp unsweetened desiccated coconut

2 tbsp cacao powder

When naming these decadent chocolate truffles, I simply had to refer to their powerful concentration of nutrients designed to target dry skin, fine lines, a dull complexion and other signs of ageing. The hemp seeds are a rich source of the essential omega-3 fats needed by every cell in your body and to keep skin soft, while the dates are a natural fibre-rich sweetener and are packed with vitamin A for healthy skin and good eyesight. The raw cacao powder is one of the best sources of antioxidants to combat the free radicals that age our faces. It also just so happens to be an aphrodisiac, so these treats are best saved for a romantic night in with that special someone!

1   Soak the dates in a small bowl of warm water for 15–20 minutes to soften. Drain well.

2   Chop the soaked dates into small pieces and place in a blender or food processor with the hemp seeds, cacao powder, cinnamon and vanilla. Blend together until a sticky dough forms. It's also possible to use a fork or potato masher for this. Roll the mixture into 10–12 small truffle-sized balls between the palms of your hands.

3   Place the coconut and the remaining 2 tablespoons of cacao powder in separate shallow bowls. Coat some of the truffles in the coconut and the remainder in the cacao powder.

4   Store the truffles in an airtight container in the fridge for up to four days.

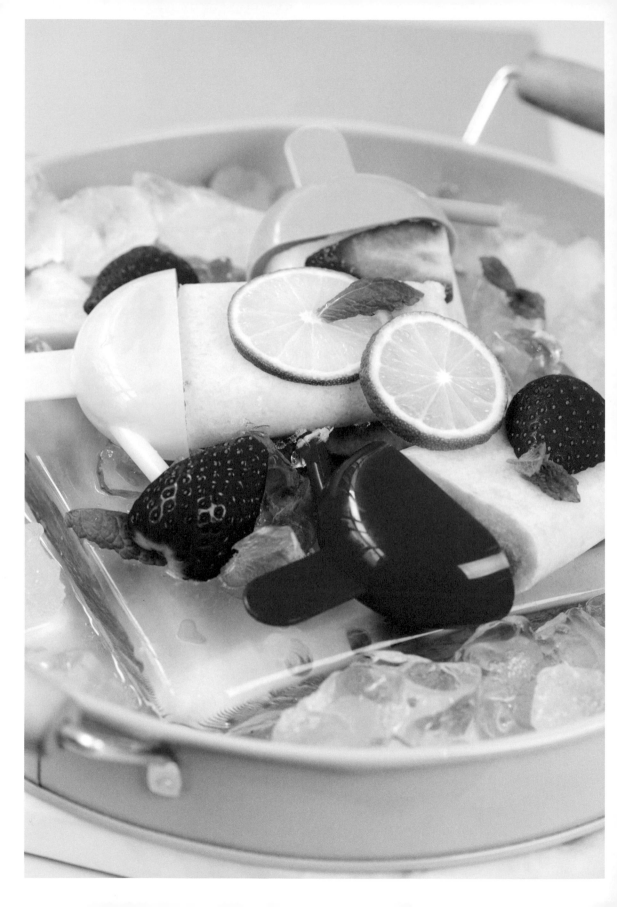

TOTALLY TROPICAL SMOOTHIE POPS

Makes 4 ice pops

170g pineapple chunks

2 ripe bananas, peeled

1 fresh mango, pitted, peeled and sliced

120ml low-fat coconut milk

My mum used to make ice pops in the summer months when I was a child, and my brothers and I loved the sweet, cold simplicity of them. They're great for kids and so easy to whizz up and freeze to cool the family down on warm days. Since tropical fruits are so summery in flavour, I've used them for this recipe.

1   Place the pineapple chunks, bananas, mangos and coconut milk in a blender and combine until very smooth. Pour into an ice pop mould, insert the ice pop sticks and put in the freezer for 4–5 hours or overnight, until frozen.
2   Briefly run hot water over the outside of the ice pop moulds to loosen them. Remove the ice pops from their moulds and serve immediately.

MAPLE AND PECAN PIE

Serves 6–8

FOR THE FILLING:

150g dates, pitted

100g chopped pecans

1 ripe banana, peeled

2 heaped tbsp chia seeds

1 tbsp ground cinnamon

2 tsp vanilla extract

$\frac{1}{2}$ tsp ground nutmeg

60g fresh blueberries, to decorate

30g whole pecans, to decorate

FOR THE CRUST:

145g ground almonds

85g pure maple syrup

55g organic virgin coconut oil

1 tsp vanilla extract

Just like all the sweet treats and desserts in this section, this maple and pecan pie must be viewed as an occasional 'cheat' food if you want to look and feel your most healthy and beautiful. While it's raw, vegan and free from refined sugar, dairy and gluten, the ingredients are still energy rich. However, this is a fantastic dessert to make for friends and family on special feast days like Christmas, Easter or birthdays. I've made this as a vegan option on Christmas Day for the past few years and it always gets polished off. Maple and pecan is a classic flavour combo, enhanced even more by the warming spices. I also like to decorate the pie with some fresh blueberries for a dash of colour and added antioxidants.

1 Soak the dates in a small bowl of warm water for 15–20 minutes to soften. Drain well.

2 Place all the ingredients for the crust into a blender or food processor and combine until a dough forms. Press firmly and evenly into a medium-sized round silicone or springform tin.

3 Place the soaked dates, chopped pecans, banana, chia seeds, cinnamon, vanilla and nutmeg into the blender or food processor and blend until smooth. Pour the filling over the crust, ensuring it's flat and even. Decorate with the blueberries and whole pecans. Be creative! Transfer to the freezer and allow it to set for at least 4 hours.

4 When ready to serve, remove the pie from the freezer and carefully cut into slices with a sharp knife. Leftovers can be stored in a sealed container in the freezer for up to three months.

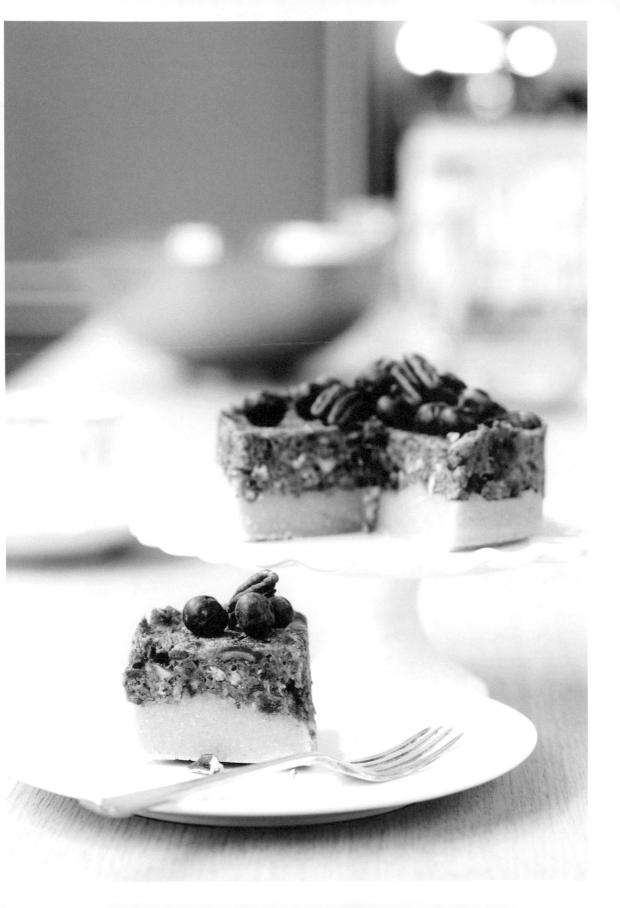

CREAMY CHOCOLATE MOUSSE

Serves 2

75g Medjool dates, pitted

1 large, ripe avocado, peeled and pitted

1 banana, peeled, chopped into chunks and frozen

60ml unsweetened almond milk

2 heaped tbsp raw cacao powder

1 tsp vanilla extract

handful of fresh raspberries, to serve

For chocoholics everywhere, a sinfully delicious chocolate mousse is one of the naughtiest desserts going. So most people look at me in disbelief when I tell them that it can be made in a way that is healthy and beneficial for our skin and body. I made this super-simple raw chocolate mousse for a group of girl-friends recently who all went back for seconds and then begged me for the recipe! The creamy avocado is an incredible food for a smooth and supple complexion, while raw cacao powder is one of the very best antioxidants in the world.

1 Soak the dates in a small bowl of warm water for 15–20 minutes to soften. Drain well.

2 Put the soaked dates in a blender or food processor and blend until they become a smooth paste. Add the avocado, frozen banana, almond milk, cacao powder and vanilla extract and blend until the mousse is smooth and creamy.

3 Spoon the mousse into two individual serving bowls and place in the fridge for 45–60 minutes, until it sets. Serve with fresh raspberries scattered on top.

RAW RASPBERRY RIPPLE CHEESECAKE

Serves 6

FOR THE FILLING:

375g cashew nuts, organic if possible

450g coconut cream

55g coconut oil, melted

juice of 1 lemon

3 tbsp pure organic maple syrup or to taste

1 tsp vanilla extract

125g frozen raspberries, thawed

FOR THE BASE:

150g dates, pitted

225g almonds

40g unsweetened desiccated coconut

1 tsp vanilla extract

TO DECORATE:

1 tbsp thawed frozen raspberries

2 tbsp cold water

125g fresh blueberries

sprig of fresh mint

My family and friends are usually surprised when I produce this amazingly vibrant raw vegan cheesecake because it looks like the real deal and tastes great but doesn't make you feel bloated or weighed down after eating it. It's still most definitely a treat food and not for everyday enjoyment, but the berries fill you with valuable antioxidants to fight fine lines, while the dates and nuts provide plenty of protein, fibre and healthy fats.

1   To make the base, soak the dates in a small bowl of warm water for 15–20 minutes to soften. Drain well.

2   Place the almonds in a blender or food processor and blend until the texture becomes crumbly. Add in the soaked dates, coconut and vanilla. Process until well combined and the mixture sticks together between your fingers. Add a little water if necessary. Spoon the mixture into the bottom of a medium-sized circular silicone or springform tin and place in the freezer to set.

3   To make the cheesecake filling, place the cashews in the blender or food processor and blend until they become crumbly. Add in the coconut cream, melted coconut oil, lemon juice, maple syrup to taste and vanilla extract and blend until smooth and creamy.

4   Remove the base from the freezer and spread half of the filling on top. Spread the thawed raspberries in a layer across the top, then cover with the rest of the filling.

5   To make the raspberry ripple, blend the tablespoon of thawed raspberries with 2 tablespoons of cold water. Spoon the ripple around the surface of the cheesecake and tease it out in swirls with a toothpick. Decorate with the fresh blueberries and mint.

6   Put the cheesecake back in the freezer to set. Remove from the freezer 15–20 minutes before serving to let it thaw slightly. This will keep in the freezer for up to three months.

COCONUT AND VANILLA STRAWBERRY SLICE

Makes 8 slices

FOR THE COCONUT AND VANILLA CREAM:

60g cashew nuts

120ml low-fat coconut milk

2 tbsp organic pure maple syrup

1 tsp vanilla extract

40g unsweetened desiccated coconut

sliced fresh strawberries, to decorate

FOR THE BASE:

75g Medjool dates, pitted

75g dried figs

50g walnuts

25g almonds

2 tbsp ground flaxseed

2 tbsp unsweetened desiccated coconut

1 tsp vanilla extract

1/2 tsp ground cinnamon

1/2 tsp cold water

This yummy raw dessert looks pretty impressive and combines three of my favourite flavours: strawberry, coconut and vanilla. I often make this for warm-weather family gatherings, like summer garden parties and barbecues, as these individual slices look so colourful and pretty arranged on a platter. People also find it difficult to believe that this dessert is healthy and free from refined sugar and processed ingredients. The healthy fats in the coconut, walnuts and almonds help to soften and rejuvenate tired-out skin, while the figs and dates do wonders for flushing excess toxins out of the body and improving digestion.

1   Soak the cashews for the filling in a small bowl of cold water for 2–3 hours, then drain. Soak the dates for the base in a small bowl of warm water for 15–20 minutes to soften. Drain well.

2   To make the base, place all the ingredients, including the soaked dates, in a food processor or blender and pulse until you can press the mixture together between your fingers and it sticks together. Pour into a 10cm x 20cm silicone tray and press down firmly with a spatula until it's even and flat. Place the tray into the freezer to set the base.

3   To make the coconut and vanilla cream, blend the cashews in the blender or food processor with a little cold water for 2 minutes. Gradually add in the coconut milk, maple syrup and vanilla extract. Continue to blend until it becomes smooth and creamy. Add in the desiccated coconut and pulse just to combine it into the mixture.

4   Remove the base from the freezer and pour the vanilla and coconut layer on top. Place the tray back into the freezer to set for 2 hours.

5   Remove the cheesecake from the freezer 15 minutes before serving to allow it to defrost slightly. Decorate with fresh strawberry slices and carefully cut into individual slices with a sharp knife. This will keep in the freezer for up to three months.

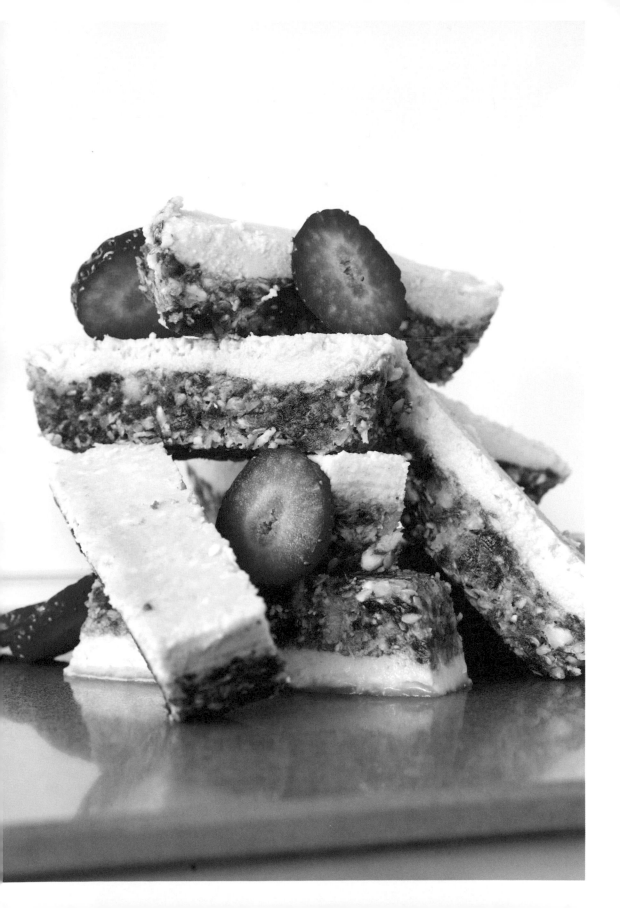

SMOOTHIES AND DRINKS

I'm a big fan of homemade smoothies and I firmly believe that they should feature in everyone's daily diet. They're such an easy way to fill your body with valuable vitamins, minerals, fibre and amino acids and require minimal digestive energy, as the nutrients are readily available to be absorbed into your blood and delivered straight to your cells. They're portable, can be prepared in large batches and frozen to save time, and the possibilities for different combinations are endless. I've selected my favourites for their range of various beauty- and health-building qualities.

Beauty tip:

AFTER A STRENUOUS WEIGHTS SESSION
IN THE GYM, I ALWAYS MAKE SURE TO
EAT A PORTION OF BERRIES FOR THEIR
ANTIOXIDANTS AND TO HELP DAMPEN DOWN
ANY POST-WORKOUT INFLAMMATION AND
MUSCLE PAIN. THE PINK WARRIOR PROTEIN
SMOOTHIE ON PAGE 223 IS A DELICIOUS
WAY TO TREAT YOUR BODY TO LOTS OF
ANTI-INFLAMMATORY NUTRIENTS. POP IN
A COUPLE TABLESPOONS OF HULLED HEMP
SEEDS OR A SCOOP OF RAW PLANT-BASED
PROTEIN POWDER TO HELP REPAIR TORN
MUSCLE FIBRES.

GREEN GODDESS SMOOTHIE

Serves 2–3

120ml cold water, to blend

200g organic baby spinach, washed well

165g pineapple chunks

125g fresh blueberries

1 ripe banana, peeled

½ organic cucumber, chopped into chunks

2 tbsp freshly squeezed lemon or lime juice

1 tbsp fresh mint leaves

1 tsp freshly grated ginger

4 ice cubes

4–5 drops of liquid stevia (optional)

This is my signature drink and one of the most important elements of the *Eat Yourself Beautiful* programme. Even if you don't make any other changes to your diet and lifestyle, simply drinking a large glass of this smoothie first thing in the morning will make a noticeable difference to your beauty, health, energy, waistline and immune system. It's that effective! I have incorporated some of the very best foods for younger-looking skin, faster hair growth, fat burning and anti-ageing into one drink. It's easy to make in big batches two or three times a week. It can be stored in the freezer or it keeps fresh in the fridge for two or three days, so there are no excuses! Drink it regularly and look forward to improved digestion and elimination, a flatter stomach, glowing skin, better protection from colds and flu and thicker hair. Plus it's far cheaper than doctor bills, prescription medicines and expensive beauty products.

1   Add the water to the blender first, followed by the spinach, pineapple, blueberries, banana, cucumber, lemon juice, mint leaves, ginger and ice cubes. Blend until smooth and creamy. Taste and add a few drops of liquid stevia if desired.

2   Serve chilled in a tall glass. You can store any leftovers in the freezer or it keeps fresh in the fridge for two or three days.

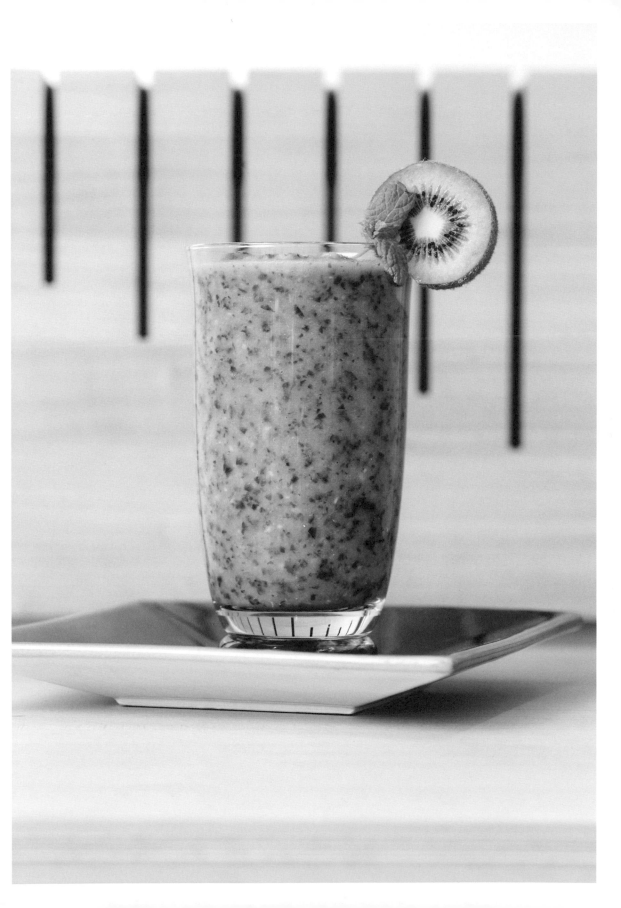

BLOAT-BANISHING ELECTROLYTE SMOOTHIE

Serves 2

300g watermelon, cut into chunks and seeds removed

2 large cooked beetroots, quartered

2 stalks of celery, cut into small pieces

1 banana, peeled, cut into chunks and frozen for 4–5 hours

250ml coconut water

4 ice cubes

4–5 drops of liquid stevia (optional)

sprig of fresh mint, to decorate

Feeling bloated and uncomfortable in your clothes or after eating is such a common occurrence and I'm often asked for my tips on how to combat it. I know that certain foods like wheat and refined salt and sugar trigger bloating with me and alcohol is another culprit, so I try to avoid them as much as I possibly can to look and feel my best. If I'm feeling a little bloated because of airplane travel or my hormones, I assemble all the very best anti-bloat foods in one big smoothie and it always works a treat. This combination of watermelon, beetroot, banana, celery and coconut water works so well because they're extremely alkalising foods, rich in potassium and other natural electrolytes, which are cleansing for blood and tissues and have a high water content. Together, they boost kidney function, balance your body's electrolytes, stimulate your lymphatic system and encourage your cells and tissues to release stored-up fluid.

1   Put the watermelon, beetroots, celery, frozen banana, coconut water and ice cubes in a blender. Process on a high speed until very smooth. Taste and add a few drops of liquid stevia if desired.

2   Serve chilled in a jar or tall glass and decorate with a sprig of fresh mint. Any leftovers will keep in the fridge in an airtight container for up to two days.

BRAIN-BOOSTING BLUEBERRY AND COCONUT SMOOTHIE

Serves 2

2 ripe bananas, peeled
125g fresh blueberries
120ml coconut water
$^1/_2$ tsp vanilla extract
4 ice cubes
desiccated coconut, to
decorate

This is one of my favourite go-to recipes when a sugar craving hits. The natural fruit sugars conquer the craving while filling you up with nutrients for body and brain, such as the vitamin B6 found in bananas, which is one of the main co-factors in producing serotonin to curb those hankerings for all foods naughty but nice! Blueberries are also a rich source of wrinkle-busting antioxidants. You shouldn't drink fruit juices too often because the fruit fibre has been removed and the sugars are absorbed immediately into your bloodstream, leading to a roller coaster of blood sugar spikes and crashes, which definitely impact mood. But this smoothie contains all of the fibre, so the natural fruit sugar is absorbed more slowly, just as nature intended.

1 Combine all the ingredients together in a blender until smooth.
2 Pour into a tall glass, decorate with desiccated coconut and serve chilled. Any leftovers will keep in the fridge in an airtight container for up to two days.

MANGO MUDDLE SMOOTHIE

Serves 2

135g fresh kale

165g mango, peeled, pitted, chopped into chunks and frozen

50g cucumber (I buy organic and leave the skin on)

½ ripe avocado, peeled and pitted

250ml coconut water

2 tbsp freshly squeezed lime juice

4 ice cubes

fresh mint leaves, to decorate

This smoothie is a great way to get children to eat their greens and I often recommend it to clients who are trying to get their family to adopt healthier food habits. The cold sweetness of the frozen mango with the tangy lime and creamy avocado manage to hide any 'green' taste from the kale and cucumber.

1   Wash the kale well and dry it in a salad spinner or pat dry with kitchen paper. Remove the tough stems and discard them.
2   Place all the ingredients in a blender and combine until smooth and creamy.
3   Pour into a tall glass, decorate with the fresh mint leaves and serve chilled. Any leftovers will keep in the fridge in an airtight container for up to two days.

PINK WARRIOR PROTEIN SMOOTHIE

Serves 2

4 organic cooked beetroots

1 ripe banana, peeled

60g fresh or frozen raspberries

60g fresh or frozen blueberries

2 scoops of Sunwarrior vanilla raw protein powder or raw hemp protein powder

120ml coconut water

4 ice cubes

1 fresh fig, sliced, to serve

1 tsp chia seeds, to serve

For ladies who lift! This is one of my favourite recovery smoothies after a tough weights workout, as the easily digested raw plant protein helps to repair torn muscle fibres, the anti-oxidants work hard against the ageing free radicals produced during a hard exercise session, the coconut water helps to rehydrate and the natural sugars boost flagging energy levels without raising them too high, as the fibre keeps it all steady. Plus the colour is really pretty!

1 Place all the ingredients in a blender and combine until smooth.

2 Pour into a tall glass and decorate with sliced figs and chia seeds. Serve cold. Any leftovers will keep in the fridge in an airtight container for up to two days.

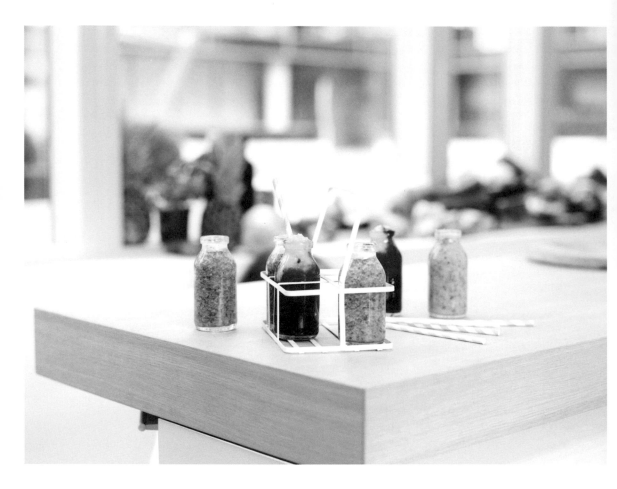

RAINBOW BERRY BLAST

Serves 2

FOR THE BOTTOM LAYER:

75g frozen blackberries

75g frozen blueberries

2–3 tbsp coconut water to blend, if necessary

FOR THE MIDDLE LAYER:

125g frozen raspberries

110g frozen strawberries

1 tsp pure vanilla extract

2–3 tbsp coconut water to blend, if necessary

FOR THE TOP LAYER:

85g mango, peeled, pitted, cut into chunks and frozen

2 bananas, peeled, cut into chunks and frozen

2–3 tbsp low-fat coconut milk

squeeze of fresh lime juice

2 fresh, ripe strawberries, sliced, to serve

This brightly coloured rainbow smoothie not only looks impressive, but it also delivers a serious antioxidant boost to brighten up tired, dull skin and protect your immune system from bugs. Serve in a glass jar to make the most of the layered berry hues.

1 Begin with the bottom layer by placing the ingredients in a blender and combining until smooth, using a few tablespoons of coconut water if necessary to help it blend. Pour it into the bottom of two glass jars, ensuring it's smooth. Place briefly in the freezer while you prepare the next layer.
2 Repeat the same process for the middle layer as you did for the base. Pour the middle layer into the jars on top of the base layer and ensure it's even. Place back in the freezer.
3 Repeat the process once more for the top layer. Pour on top of the middle layer, decorate with sliced strawberries and serve immediately. Any leftovers will keep in the fridge in an airtight container for up to two days.

CHOCOLATE CHIP
THICKSHAKE

Serves 2

250ml unsweetened
almond milk

4 bananas, peeled, chopped
and frozen for 4–5 hours

4 Medjool dates, pitted

2 scoops of Sunwarrior raw
vegan chocolate protein
powder (optional)

2 heaped tbsp raw cacao
powder

2 tbsp raw cacao nibs,
plus extra to decorate

2 tsp pure vanilla extract

4 ice cubes

Craving something chocolaty and satisfying? This is one seriously thick and creamy smoothie, but it's not nearly as naughty as the name suggests! The all-natural ingredients in this shake will quench any craving for something sweet and cold, but it's brimming with beauty-building nutrients and none of the ageing refined sugar, unhealthy fats and other chemical ingredients in your typical chocolate milkshake. Hurrah!

1   Put all the ingredients in a blender and blend until smooth and creamy. Add a little more almond milk if a thinner consistency is desired.

2   Pour into a tall glass, decorate with a sprinkle of cacao nibs and serve chilled. Any leftovers will keep in the fridge in an airtight container for up to two days.

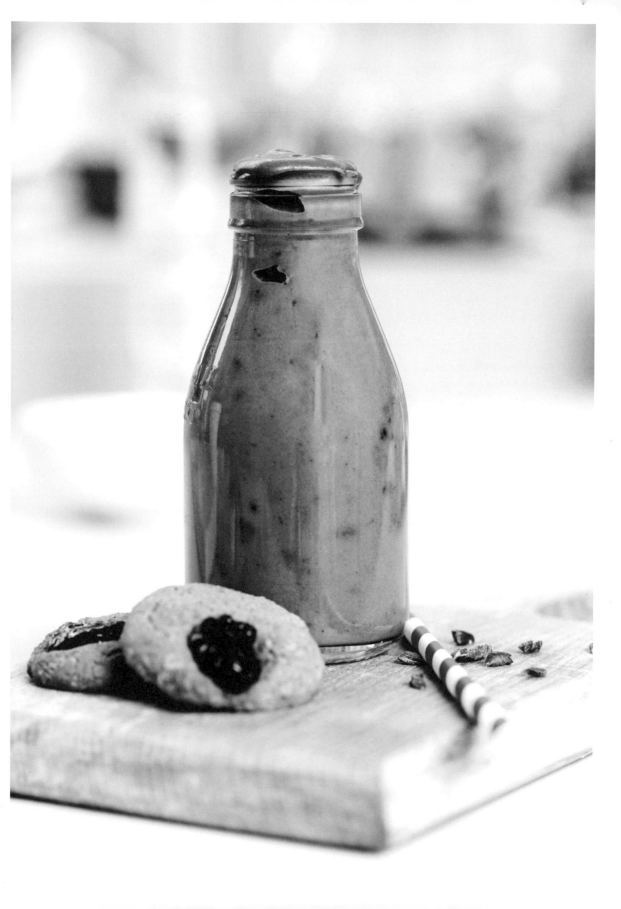

GREEN MACHINE
HERBAL CLEANSER

Serves 2

250ml coconut water

1 green apple, cored
and halved

¹/₂ avocado, peeled and pitted

80g fresh pineapple

50g cucumber

30g baby spinach, rinsed well

15g fresh flat-leaf parsley

2 tbsp chopped fresh mint

2 tbsp freshly squeezed
lime juice

4 ice cubes

2 slices of fresh kiwi, to serve

We all need to be eating more greens, ideally at every meal because they're the most nutrient-dense type of food there is. They will help you to reach your health, beauty and weight goals better than any other food. This green smoothie is packed with blood- and cell-cleansing greens, plus the sweeter flavours of green apple, pineapple and lime balance it all out.

1 Place all the ingredients in a blender and combine until smooth.
2 Pour into a tall glass, decorate with kiwi slices and serve chilled. Any leftovers will keep in the fridge in an airtight container for up to two days.

HORMONE-BALANCING CHIA AND CINNAMON THICKSHAKE

Serves 2

500ml unsweetened almond milk

2 bananas, peeled, chopped and frozen

2 Medjool dates, pitted

2 scoops of Sunwarrior vanilla vegan protein powder

2 heaped tbsp maca powder

2 tbsp chia seeds

1 tbsp raw organic coconut oil

2 tsp ground cinnamon, plus extra to serve

2 tsp pure vanilla extract

4 ice cubes

Ladies, if you have ever suffered the crippling pain of menstrual cramps, you'll know exactly how excruciating and debilitating it can be. I used to really suffer and would sometimes spend the entire day in bed curled around a hot water bottle with pain and nausea. It was only when I began to focus on balancing my hormones naturally, loaded up on omega-3 fats and decreased the amounts of omega-6 fats I was eating in vegetable oils and animal-based foods that I found relief. In fact, it made such an enormous difference that I barely feel anything these days and life can go on as normal. I designed this shake to fill you up with anti-inflammatory fats, plenty of fibre and the hormone-balancing benefits of maca powder. A tuber similar to a radish, maca helps to stabilise your hormones naturally and supports your adrenals, plus it's rich in amino acids, calcium, potassium, iron, magnesium, phosphorus and zinc.

Note: Do not take maca during pregnancy.

1   Place all the ingredients in a blender and combine on a high speed until smooth and creamy.
2   Pour into a tall glass, decorate with a sprinkle of cinnamon and serve chilled. Any leftovers will keep in the fridge in an airtight container for up to two days.

STRAWBERRIES AND CREAM SUMMER PROTEIN SHAKE

Serves 2

150g frozen strawberries (make sure to rinse them well before freezing)

1 ripe banana, peeled, cut into chunks and frozen for 4-5 hours

250ml low-fat coconut milk (or coconut milk yoghurt for a creamier shake)

120ml coconut water

2 scoops of Sunwarrior vanilla protein powder

2 tsp vanilla extract

4 ice cubes

2 large, ripe strawberries, sliced, to serve

It's hard to beat the taste of summer's first juicy strawberries. As a child, my mum used to prepare us big bowls of strawberries and cream to enjoy sitting in the sunshine outside in the garden and this smoothie brings me right back. It makes a great snack or filling breakfast, especially if you use coconut milk yoghurt as the base.

1   Put all the ingredients in a blender and combine on high speed until smooth and creamy.
2   Pour into two glasses and decorate with strawberry slices. Serve chilled.

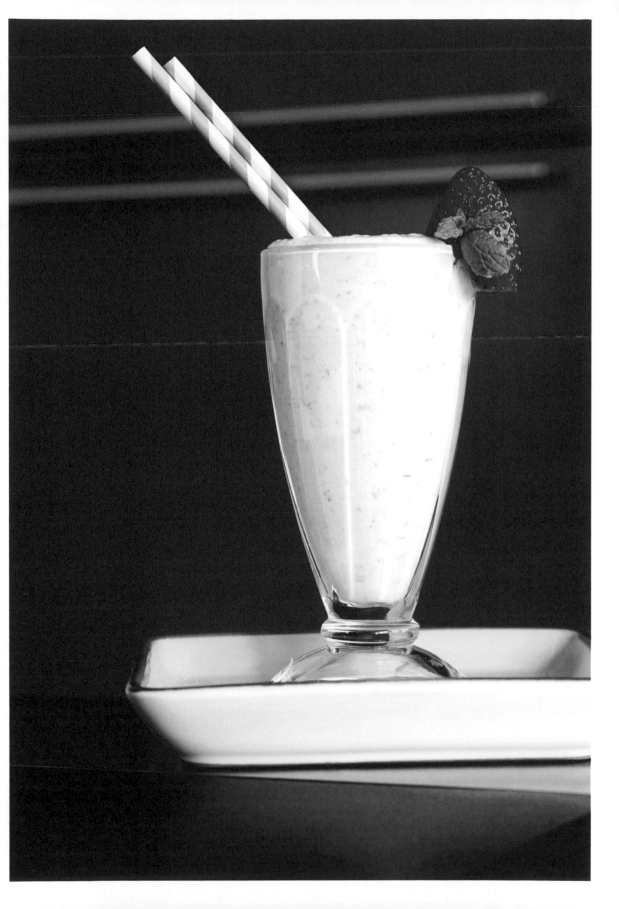

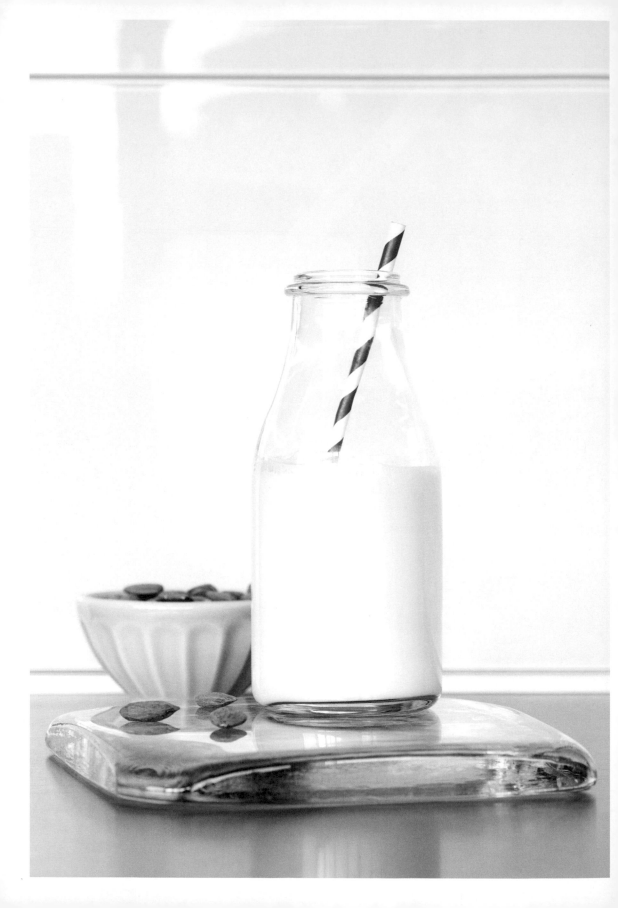

HOMEMADE ALMOND MILK

Makes 500ml

150g whole almonds (organic if possible)

500ml cold water

2 Medjool dates, pitted (optional)

2 tbsp pure maple syrup (optional)

2 tsp pure vanilla extract (optional)

Some brands of commercial almond milk can be full of added sugar and toxic thickeners like carrageenan, which is why it's important to be aware when choosing which one to buy. However, homemade almond milk is surprisingly easy and inexpensive to make at home, is totally natural and can be adapted to your own individual taste. As it lasts in the fridge for only two days in an airtight container, I only tend to make as much as I think I'll use. It's so delicious poured over porridge and in chia pudding recipes and it makes my homemade healthy hot chocolate recipe on page 234 irresistibly smooth and creamy.

1   Soak the almonds for 8 hours or overnight in a bowl of cold water. Make sure the almonds are covered by at least 2.5cm of water, as they will absorb some of the liquid and expand. Drain and rinse the almonds. They should feel quite soft.

2   Place the almonds in a blender with the cold water and blend on a high speed for at least 2 minutes, until the almonds have been ground down finely and the water has turned milky. Taste it and add your chosen sweetener, if desired.

3   Using a cheesecloth or a clean piece of muslin, strain the almond milk into a jug or large jar. Squeeze the cloth to ensure all the milk has drained out and only the almond meal remains. Store in an airtight container in the fridge for up to two days.

CINNAMON-SPICED HOT CHOCOLATE

Serves 2

500ml unsweetened
almond milk

3 heaped tbsp raw cacao
powder, plus extra to serve

1 tsp ground cinnamon

liquid stevia

1 tsp coconut sugar

Sometimes all I crave on dark evenings is a big, warming mug of hot chocolate. But there's no need to sabotage your healthy eating plan with sugar-laden commercial varieties when healthy, nourishing hot chocolate is so simple to make. The raw cacao powder is brimming with antioxidants, while the cinnamon aids blood sugar control. I make this recipe at least twice a week in the wintertime. I use a milk-frothing device to make the almond milk really thick and foamy, but it works just as well without one.

1   Boil a kettle of water.
2   Warm up the almond milk in a small saucepan over a medium heat until it almost boils. Remove from the heat.
3   Place 1 ½ tablespoons of cacao powder and ½ teaspoon of cinnamon into each of two separate mugs. Pour in the boiled water, filling each cup by one-third. Stir the cacao powder and cinnamon until they are evenly dissolved in the water. Add four or five drops of liquid stevia to each cup to sweeten it if desired.
4   Froth up the almond milk until it reaches your desired consistency and pour into each mug. Stir gently. Top each mug with a pinch of cacao powder and ½ teaspoon of coconut sugar. Serve while hot.

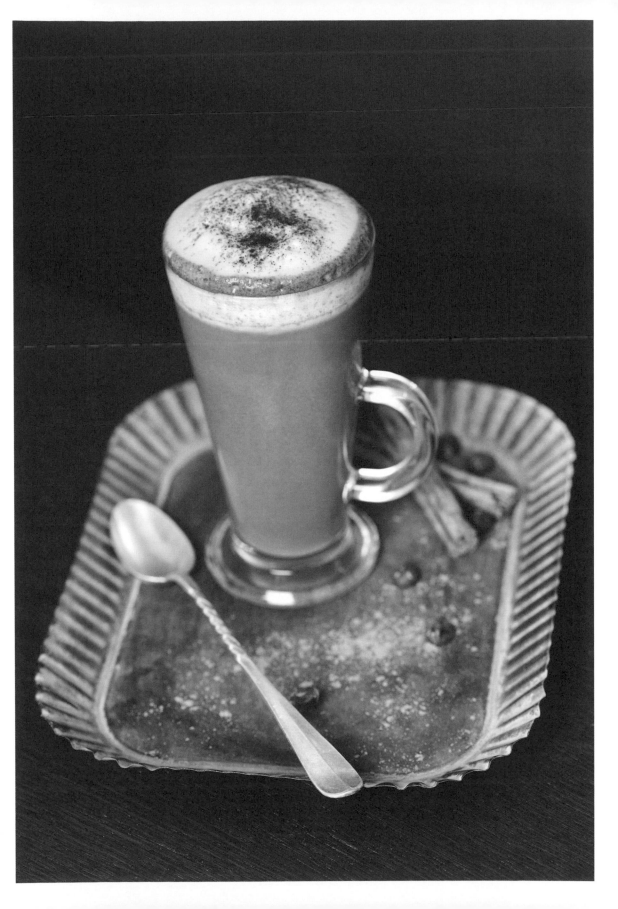

BEAUTY SNACKS

These are some of my favourite snacks to grab when on the go,
travelling or after a workout to keep me going until the next meal.
They're all simple, quick and nourishing for your skin,
hair and body.

Beauty tip:

FATS ARE ESSENTIAL FOR BEAUTIFUL, SOFT
SKIN AND A YOUTHFUL COMPLEXION.
AVOCADOS ARE ONE OF THE MOST SUPERIOR
FOODS YOU CAN EAT FOR THEIR HEALTHY
FATS AND AMAZING BEAUTY BENEFITS, SO
THEY FEATURE HIGHLY ON MY LIST OF TOP
SKIN FOODS. AIM TO EAT ABOUT HALF AN
AVOCADO A DAY WITH YOUR MEALS, OR AS
A SNACK WITH CRUNCHY VEGGIES DIPPED
INTO FRESHLY MADE GUACAMOLE.

OMEGA-3 KALE CRISPS

Serves 2

coconut oil, for greasing

1 bag of curly kale

2 medium, ripe tomatoes

1 red pepper, deseeded

1 clove of garlic, peeled

juice of 1/2 lime

4 tbsp nutritional yeast (I sprinkle a little more onto the kale before it goes into the dehydrator or oven)

3 tbsp hulled hemp seeds

2 tbsp apple cider vinegar

2 tbsp Bragg Liquid Amino or low-sodium tamari sauce

pinch of chilli flakes

freshly ground black pepper

I'm obsessed with kale crisps, a crispy, crunchy and thoroughly guilt-free alternative to regular crisps. I'm lucky enough to own a dehydrator, which heats food just enough without destroying the delicate nutrients. If you don't have one, then these will dehydrate well in an oven on a low temperature with the door left open. Kale is a true star veggie as it boasts more calcium than milk, more iron than beef, 10% more vitamin C than spinach and is high in antioxidants, vitamins and minerals for superior health and beauty, plus plenty of fibre to help clear toxins from your body. It's the goody two-shoes of the veggie world! And this snack is a truly delicious and easy way to enjoy kale. In this recipe, I use hulled hemp seeds, which are an amazing source of omega-3 fats and easily digested plant protein. Two tablespoons contain 5 grams of protein, plus essential minerals including iron, zinc, phosphorus and magnesium. These crisps are pretty much a perfect food!

1   Preheat the oven to 160°C. Lightly grease a baking tray with coconut oil if you are using an oven.
2   Wash the kale and pat it dry before breaking it into smaller pieces and removing the hard, thick stems. Put the kale in a large bowl.
3   Blend the tomatoes, red pepper, garlic, lime juice, nutritional yeast, hemp seeds, apple cider vinegar, liquid aminos, a pinch of chilli flakes and some freshly ground black pepper in a blender or food processor until smooth.
4   Pour the dressing over the kale and mix together well, then spread the kale out on the greased baking tray if using an oven. If using a dehydrator, spread the kale out on the trays, close it and set the dial to the pre-set temperature for vegetables.
5   Bake for 15–20 minutes with the oven door open. Keep a close eye on the crisps, as they burn easily. Remove as soon as they're crispy and serve straightaway. The crisps can be stored in an airtight container for up to three days but they can lose their crispiness.

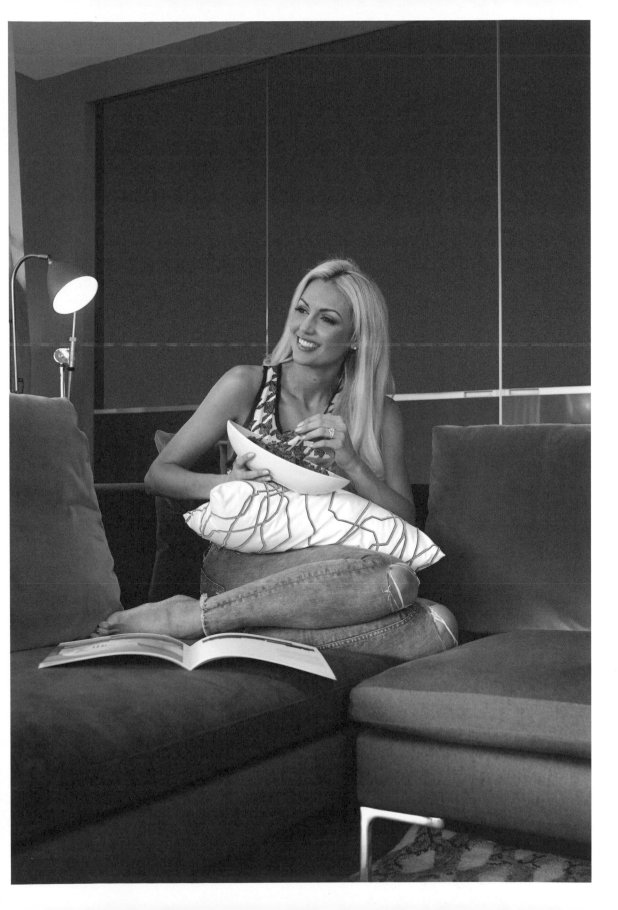

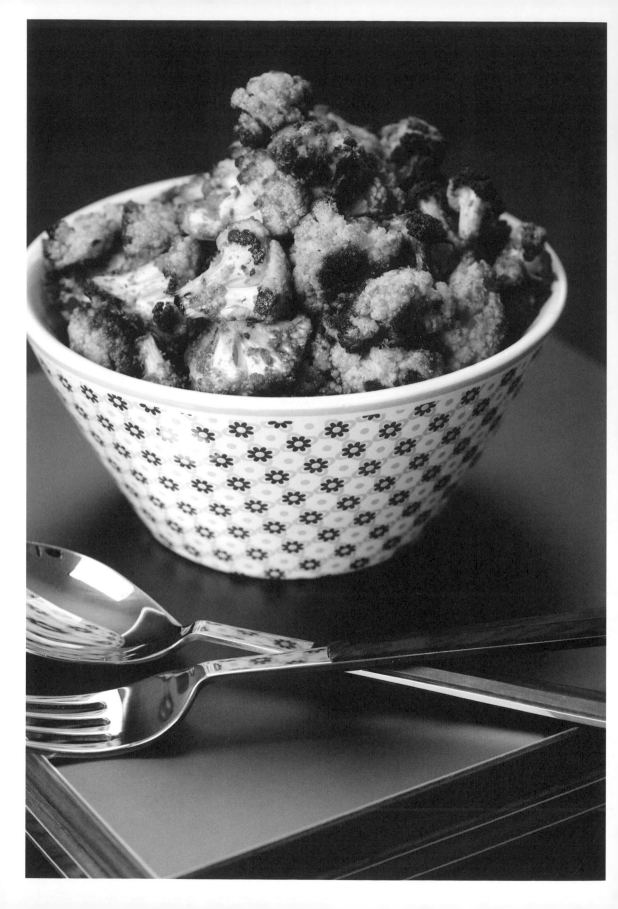

CHEESY TURMERIC
CAULI BITES

Serves 2

2 heaped tbsp nutritional yeast, plus extra for sprinkling

2 tbsp freshly squeezed lemon juice

2 tsp melted organic virgin coconut oil, plus extra for greasing

1 tsp ground turmeric

$1/_2$ tsp smoked paprika

pinch of cayenne pepper (optional)

3-4 drops of liquid stevia

Himalayan pink rock salt and freshly ground black pepper

1 medium head of cauliflower, chopped into small bite-sized pieces

Turmeric is truly a superstar spice. It has been used for centuries for its anti-inflammatory and skin-brightening benefits, so I'm always looking for inventive ways to include more of it in my diet. I really love these cheesy turmeric cauli bites as a simple snack, but also for cauliflower's many health benefits. These bites are a little bit like popcorn, but of course without the rivers of melted butter and salt. I use mineral-rich nutritional yeast to give them a cheesy flavour. Try them the next time you sit down to a movie or box set at home. They're the perfect, healthy TV snack.

1   Preheat the oven to 190°C. Lightly grease a baking tray with coconut oil.

2   In a big mixing bowl, stir together the nutritional yeast, lemon juice, coconut oil, turmeric, smoked paprika, a pinch of cayenne pepper (if using), a few drops of liquid stevia and some salt and pepper. Add the cauliflower pieces and mix together well to ensure that each piece is liberally covered in the spices.

3   Spread the coated cauli bites out on the greased tray. Sprinkle a little more nutritional yeast on top.

4   Cook in the oven for 10 minutes. Turn the florets over and cook for 5 minutes more to allow the pieces to turn golden brown and crispy. Serve straightaway while still warm.

BEDTIME BANANA BITES

Serves 2

2 medium, ripe bananas, peeled

pinch of ground cinnamon

FOR THE ALMOND BUTTER:

675g unsalted almonds

2 tsp pure organic vanilla extract

There is no need to splash out on pricey shop-bought almond butter when it's so simple to make at home. All you need are raw almonds and a little patience, as it can be a time-consuming process waiting for the nuts to transform into almond butter. But it's so worth it! That's why I tend to make it in bigger batches and store it in the fridge to use over a few days. Almond butter can be used and enjoyed in multiple ways, but I really love these vanilla almond butter banana bites as an evening snack about an hour before I go to bed. They can help to induce sleep because the almond butter is a good source of tryptophan and the bananas are full of vitamin B6. Both are necessary to make your sleep hormone, melatonin, to help you peacefully drift off.

1 To make the almond butter, place the almonds in a blender or food processor and blend for 20–30 minutes, stopping frequently to scrape down the sides. Use a splash of water if necessary to help it blend. The almonds will eventually release their natural oils, which results in a butter with a smooth and creamy texture. Once smooth, add the vanilla extract.

2 This makes about 375g, so spoon the leftover almond butter into a jar and store in the fridge for up to five days.

3 Slice the bananas and set them on a large plate. Spread a teaspoon of the almond butter on every second slice and top with the plain slice, creating a sandwich. Sprinkle with a dusting of cinnamon and serve straightaway.

FUNKY TRAIL MIX

unsalted almonds
walnut halves
sunflower seeds
pumpkin seeds
unsweetened coconut flakes
unsweetened dried
cranberries
dried goji berries

A version of trail mix comes with me on almost every short airplane journey I take because it's so convenient and versatile. On long-haul flights I'll always order a vegan meal, but on short hops it's often difficult to get hold of something healthy, so all of this essential fat and fibre keeps me going until I can get a proper meal. I use a sealable clear sandwich bag and pop in a small handful of each of the ingredients listed.

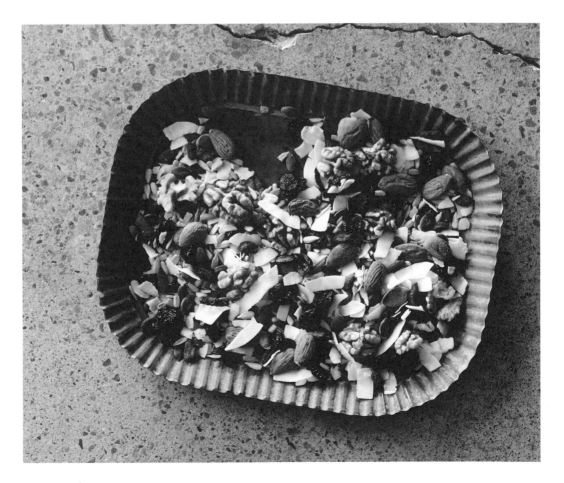

INDEX